a–z of health promotion

Professional Keywords series

Every field of practice has its own methods, terminology, conceptual debates and landmark publications. The *Professional Keywords* series expertly structures this material into easy-reference A to Z format. Focusing on the ideas and themes that shape the field, and informed by the latest research, these books are designed both to guide the student reader and to refresh practitioners' thinking and understanding.

Available now

Mark Doel and Timothy B. Kelly: *A–Z of Groups & Groupwork*
Jon Glasby and Helen Dickinson: *A–Z of Interagency Working*
Richard Hugman: *A–Z of Professional Ethics*
Glenn Laverack: *A–Z of Health Promotion*
Neil McKeganey: *A–Z of Addiction and Substance Misuse*
Steve Nolan and Margaret Holloway: *A–Z of Spirituality*
Marian Roberts: *A–Z of Mediation*

Available soon

Jane Dalrymple: *A–Z of Advocacy*
David Shemmings, Yvonne Shemmings and David Wilkins:
    A–Z of Attachment Theory
Jeffrey Longhofer: *A–Z of Psychodynamic Practice*
David Garnett: *A–Z of Housing*
Fiona Timmins: *A–Z of Reflective Practice*

a–z of

health
promotion

Glenn Laverack

palgrave
macmillan

First published 2014 by
PALGRAVE MACMILLAN

Palgrave Macmillan in the UK is an imprint of Macmillan Publishers Limited, registered in England, company number 785998, of Houndmills, Basingstoke, Hampshire RG21 6XS.

Palgrave Macmillan in the US is a division of St Martin's Press LLC, 175 Fifth Avenue, New York, NY 10010.

Palgrave Macmillan is the global academic imprint of the above companies and has companies and representatives throughout the world.

Palgrave® and Macmillan® are registered trademarks in the United States, the United Kingdom, Europe and other countries

ISBN: 978–1–137–35048–0

This book is printed on paper suitable for recycling and made from fully managed and sustained forest sources. Logging, pulping and manufacturing processes are expected to conform to the environmental regulations of the country of origin.

A catalogue record for this book is available from the British Library.

A catalog record for this book is available from the Library of Congress.

Printed in China

contents

acknowledgements

I would like to acknowledge the many people with whom I have had the privilege of working during the course of writing this book.

Most of all my gratitude goes to my wife Elizabeth and to our three loving children Ben, Holly and Rebecca for their continued support.

how to use this book

This is a 'one-stop' source book covering a range of entries that apply to anyone working in health promotion or in associated disciplines such as public health and nursing. The writing is purposefully accessible to undergraduates and practitioners, theoretically well informed and uses empirical research, case studies and other examples sourced from the author's own experience. Additional material from the grey literature or systematically collected evidence by others, such as internet sites and data bases, is all clearly cited and referenced to indicate the relative strength of the information that is presented.

Each of the 72 main entries is written to provide sufficient reference information on a particular subject or a place-holder heading to direct the reader to a populated entry. The book does not have to be read sequentially as the reader can access any one entry, or any combination of entries, separately. Other useful features include the use of systematic italicized cross-referencing embedded in the narrative and 'see also' references under each entry to aid navigability and encourage readers to move from one entry to another. A list of contents and a detailed index also assist ease of access along a pathway that reflects the reader's own interests and needs. Each entry has a listing of up to three key texts, websites and further sources of information to encourage the reader to gain a more in-depth understanding of the subject area.

It is recommended that the reader first chooses an entry listed in the list of contents, or in the index of the book, that matches the term about which they wish to gain a better understanding. For example, the entry *theory and models* will provide the student with a good understanding of the theoretical foundations of health promotion. Alternatively, the entry *social marketing* will provide the practitioner with an understanding of a methodology commonly used in health promotion programmes. Each entry has been written to provide the reader with a precise definition, a theoretical and, where appropriate, a historical background. For entries with a practical purpose, some examples of application have been provided in a programme context. If the reader requires further information, they can simply follow the 'see also' references under each heading to aid navigability or consult one of the key texts, websites and further sources listed at the end of the entry.

introduction

Whilst there is no singularly accepted definition of health promotion, its operational purpose, formalized by both the Ottawa and Bangkok Charters, is generally agreed to be 'enabling people to increase control-over, and to improve, their health, and its determinants' (WHO, 1986; WHO, 2005). In practice, much of the work that health promoters do is intended to help others to increase their level of control-over their lives, health and its determinants. The A–Z of health promotion has been specifically written with this empowering purpose in mind.

Health promotion often includes the use of more than one model on which its practice is based, and this presents the challenge of how to apply the correct theory (the science) within the appropriate practice context (the art). Health promoters continually have to shift their attention between theory and practice and across the broader professional arena. This creates specific challenges such as linking theory and practice, identifying the evidence base, defining concepts and establishing guiding principles. A specific professional need that this book meets is to provide a comprehensive source of reference to better inform the application of the theory in the achievement of health promotion best practice.

Within health promotion, there is always some power relationship, primarily between the practitioner and their clients. Health promotion practitioners are employed to deliver information, resources and services set within the design of an intervention, a project or a programme. The practitioner is employed by a government department, agency or government-funded non-governmental organization and is often seen as an outside agent by their clients. Practitioners call themselves 'health promoters' or 'public health workers', while many more who look to the idea of health promotion occupy roles such as nurses, social workers and doctors. Their 'clients' cover the range of people with whom they work including patients, women, adolescents, men and other professional groups. The terms 'practitioner' and 'client' have been intentionally used in this book because they help to demonstrate the unbalanced power relationship that often exists in health promotion.

This book has been written to offer a convenient means to access and quickly understand the many terms, definitions and concepts used in health promotion theory and practice. I believe that this book will provide a unique and invaluable companion to students and professionals. To anyone who is interested in and passionate about promoting health, and enabling others to gain more control over its determinants, this book is a definitive source of reference.

a

advocacy

SEE ALSO competencies; declarations and statements; empowerment; media

Advocacy involves people acting on behalf of themselves or on behalf of others to argue a position and to influence the outcome of decisions. In health promotion practice, advocacy initiatives are usually started to support particular causes, interest groups and ideologies (Smithies and Webster, 1998).

The Ottawa Charter for health promotion states that actions aim at making conditions favourable for better health through advocacy (WHO, 1986). Advocacy uses both direct and indirect actions and can include *media* campaigns, public speaking and research with the intention of influencing policy, resource allocation and decision making within political and social systems.

Some of the key forms of advocacy include the following:

- Health Advocacy supports and promotes health care rights as well as enhancing *community* health and policy initiatives, for example, the availability, safety and quality of care. It focuses on education and relies on expert knowledge rather than inserting lay knowledge into expert systems (Brown *et al.*, 2004).
- Media advocacy is the strategic use of the mass media as a resource to advance a social or public policy initiative and aims to influence the selection, framing and debate of specific topics by the mass media. The goal of media advocacy is to get the media's attention and to frame the problem and solution in an appropriate way so that policy makers, politicians and the public understand the issue. Media advocacy targets the ways in which issues come to be regarded as newsworthy to help set the debate and to try to influence the boundaries within which it can take place (Wallack *et al.*, 1993).

- Collective or mass advocacy occurs when groups and organizations campaign on issues that are important to their members and who then speak out for themselves or influence what others say in the campaign, for example, through protests (Loue, Lloyd and O'Shea, 2003).
- Peer advocacy occurs when a person agrees to act on the behalf of another, for example, volunteers who are recruited to act on behalf of service users at a citizens' advice bureau.
- Self-advocacy occurs when individuals or groups share the same concerns or act on their own behalf.
- Legal advocacy occurs when a legally qualified person is employed to act on the behalf of others as an advocate, solicitor or barrister (Smithies and Webster, 1998).

In practice, the different forms of advocacy can overlap, for example, self-advocacy groups can play an important role for supporting peer advocacy and collective advocacy can support the efforts of self-advocacy groups. Action on Smoking and Health (ASH), for example, is the name of a number of autonomous advocacy groups throughout the world that has been successful in taking action against the risks associated with tobacco smoking. ASH does not blame smokers or condemn smoking but instead uses an evidence-based dual approach: information and networking and advocacy and campaigning. ASH is a campaigning health charity that also uses tactics for political influence through the creation of alliances and coalitions. ASH has had some success, for example, in 2007; it won its campaign for a total ban of smoking in enclosed public places in England including bars and private members clubs, as well as cafés, restaurants and workplaces. A similar ban is also in force in Scotland and Wales and in a number of other European countries (ASH, 2012). ASH purposefully uses indirect strategies because its status as a charity creates a dependence on funding sources including from the government.

There is a real risk that advocating on behalf of others, especially the socially marginalized, so that they are included into the economic mainstream, does not challenge the economic mainstream as being inherently socially marginalizing. For some, advocacy is ineffectual as an approach, one that does not challenge those in authority to force them to make the system more equitable.

Health promotion must do more than helping others to speak and act on their own behalf through advocacy (Labonte and Laverack, 2008). It is *empowerment* that enables others to take more control of their lives, usually through forcing social and political change. Strategies that include advocacy must therefore also use an empowerment approach for health promotion to achieve improvements in the lives and health of others.

KEY TEXTS

- Loue, S., Lloyd, L.S. and O'Shea, D.J. (2003) *Community Health Advocacy* (New York: Kluwer Academic/Plenum Publishers)
- Lustig, S. (2012) *Advocacy Strategies for Health and Mental Health Professionals: From Patients to Policies* (New York: Springer Publishing Company)
- Wallack, L.M. *et al.* (1993) *Media Advocacy and Public Health* (London: Sage Publications)

alliances, partnerships and coalitions

SEE ALSO **bottom-up and top-down; community-based intervention; civil society; networks**

An alliance is a relationship between two or more parties (individuals, groups, communities or organizations) to pursue a set of agreed upon goals, while remaining independent. The main purpose is to enable themselves, or that of others, to increase control over their lives and to improve health, going beyond health care (Jones, Sidell and Douglas, 2002). Members of the alliance provide different resources such as funding, equipment, knowledge, technology transfer, expertise or intellectual property. An alliance is therefore a collaboration that aims for a synergy where each partner's benefits are greater than those from their individual efforts. For example, to avoid facing unheated homes in the United Kingdom in winter, some communities have created alliances to purchase heating oil at cheaper prices and this has had a mutual cost benefit to all members. Alliances have two-way benefits, are participatory and in health promotion agencies do not merely consult with people but fully engage others in decision making. The structure and function of partnerships and coalitions overlap with alliances, although each has its own distinct characteristics (Laverack, 2013).

Partnerships demonstrate the ability to develop relationships with different organizations to collaborate and cooperate and to promote a heightened inter-dependency among its members. They may involve an exchange of services, pursuit of a joint venture based on a shared goal or an *advocacy* initiative to change policy. The purpose of a partnership is to grow beyond local concerns and to take a stronger position on broader issues through networking and resource mobilization. A key issue is that the members of the partnership are able to remain focused on the shared concern that brings them together, and not on the different individual needs in the partnership (Laverack, 2004).

Partnerships are an increasingly invoked strategy in health promotion. The constellation of health promotion partnerships that have been created over the past twenty years includes healthy cities/healthy communities, school, workplace, prison and other *settings* and local pilot projects such as the UK and New Zealand's Health Action Zones. A few generic lessons from using partnerships in health promotion do recur and can be summarized as follows:

- **A problem that cannot be fixed by any one group or sector.** Many partnership forums are simply information-exchanging *networks* that, while helpful in a limited way, are a questionable use of both government and *community* resources. The financial, logistical and time costs of effective partnerships can be quite large and engaging across sectors should be done with careful forethought and clarity of purpose.
- **Partners with compatible motives for action.** Ensuring that partners have overlapping interests in the problem is basic to establishing some principled action. While an argument can be made that fundamental values must also be shared, partnerships can sometimes be narrowly strategic. This brings together groups that may not hold to the same vision.
- **Partners with the resources necessary to resolve the problem.** Resources do not always have to be financial, for many community participants in partnerships that involve state sectors and NGOs, the resources they bring to the table are primarily intimate knowledge of the causes and consequences of the 'problem' that the partnership formed to resolve. However,

for some a defining feature of partnerships is the willingness of members to pool resources, primarily finances, for new initiatives.

- **Partnerships with community organizations need to be thought of as strategic alliances rather than merged identities.** Community groups pursue their own interests using their rights as citizens to make claims upon the state. Health promoters support their claims 'inside the system' through reports, advocacy and by providing an evidence base for policy analyses. However, there is a risk in many partnership activities, especially those where new service provision is one of the driving outcomes and of unintentionally transforming community activists into volunteer bureaucrats (Labonte and Laverack, 2008).

The defining characteristic of a coalition is that, by uniting around an issue, different groups can better enable their particular causes to be presented as a broad issue rather than each group's narrow interests. Coalitions tend to be temporary arrangements that form to work around one specific issue by different organizations, even though they may oppose one another on other issues. As long as the end goal is shared, however, they can set aside their differences to work cooperatively. The larger the coalition, the more likely the goal is to be achieved because the members are better able to pool their resources and to argue more persuasively in order to maximize the impact of their campaign. In other words, policymakers are more likely to listen favourably to the views of a coalition rather than similar views expressed by a number of smaller groups separately. Groups that do not commonly work together, but nevertheless find it possible to co-operate on a particular issue by itself, can suggest that the objective represents 'worthwhile' policy consideration. Decision makers are able to communicate and negotiate efficiently with a coalition by minimizing the confusion that can result from a number of groups, each *lobbying* individually on the same issue. A coalition can ensure that this level of negotiation and compromise is undertaken internally before policymakers are approached externally. Given that most coalitions are temporary arrangements focused on the achievement of limited goals, they have the potential to be relatively flexible. Successful coalitions are those that remain small and manageable and are able to both engage with community and involve its members in the development of future initiatives (McGrath, 2007).

Alliances, partnerships and coalitions are advantageous to health promotion programmes because they create shared values and collective goals, can act as a 'common voice', lead to the sharing and dissemination of information, reduce feelings of isolation, help with problem solving and reduce the duplication of efforts (Kumpfer *et al.*, 1993).

Alliances, partnerships and coalitions also assist health promotion practice because they provide a pivotal point at which the practitioner can engage with others to help them to increase control over a range of issues related to their lives, including their health and its determinants.

KEY TEXTS
- Butterfoss, D. (2007) *Coalitions and Partnerships in Community Health* (San Francisco, CA: Jossey-Bass)
- McGrath, C. (2007) 'Coalition building' in G.L. Andersen and K.G. Herr (eds), *Encyclopedia of Activism and Social Justice* (London: Sage Publications)
- Roberts, J.M. (2004) *Alliances, Coalitions and Partnerships: Building Collaborative Organisations* (Gabriola Island, Canada: New Society Publishers)

approaches

SEE ALSO **disease prevention; hegemonic power; lifespan approach; lifestyle approach; settings; theory and models**

Health promotion approaches help to better understand the different ways of working in practice as it is unlikely that any one theory or model can be applied to fulfil the requirements of a programme (Naidoo and Wills, 2009).

There are a number of different approaches to health promotion that are historically based, sometimes contradictory, and without any one being dominant or sufficient to meet the requirements of present practice. The most commonly used approaches include the medical approach, the behavioural approach, the educational approach, the client centred approach, the socio-environmental approach, the ecological approach and the *settings* approach (Naidoo and Wills, 2009).

Four inter-linked approaches that are especially relevant to shaping the way in which programmes are designed, implemented and evaluated are the medical, the behavioural, the socio-environmental and the ecological approach (the settings approach is provided in a separate entry). These approaches largely determine the strategies, the outcomes and the *evaluation* criteria that practitioners use in programme implementation. The development of these approaches in recent decades has resulted not only from the changes in our scientific understanding of health determinants and *risk factors*, but also from a growing pressure from individuals, groups and movements concerned with the health impacts of social and environmental conditions (Laverack, 2004). In health promotion practice today, some element of these different approaches are utilized in programme design. However, the following questions can help to differentiate between them: Is health promotion about improving medical treatment (medical approach)? Is health promotion about changing lifestyles (*lifestyle approach*)? Is health promotion about changing social conditions (socio-environmental approach)? (Raphael, 2000) Is health promotion about addressing the interaction of culture with environment (Ecological approach)?

It is important to appreciate how these three approaches have evolved overtime and why they have become an important part of health promotion practice, as follows.

The medical approach

Despite the evolution of competing approaches, it is the medical approach that remains dominant, socially and within health bureaucracies. This approach evolved as a result of scientific discoveries and technological advances in the 18th and 19th centuries and a greater understanding of the structure and functioning of the human body. As knowledge increased, the body became viewed as a machine that needed to be fixed; a professional split between the body and its physical illness and the condition of the mind and psyche. The focus remained on the external causes of ill health and was reinforced by the constant threat of disease and death, particularly to children, from epidemics such as polio and scarlet fever.

The medical profession established itself in the dominant position and other health professions modelled themselves on this approach to gain legitimacy including nursing, physiotherapy and, until recently, health promotion.

The medical approach is primarily concerned with the absence of disease and the treatment of illness. More recently, it has become concerned with *disease prevention* among high-risk individuals, those persons whose genetic pre-disposition, behaviour or family and personal history place them at statistically greater risk of disease. Disease prevention programmes in the medical approach are usually delivered top-down and are based on the expert (professional) knowledge. By the 1970s, a growing body of new knowledge and pressure from social movements had challenged the dominance of the medical approach, and this had led to a broadening of health knowledge to include a variety of social, behavioural and lifestyle factors (Laverack, 2004).

The behavioural/lifestyle approach

Lifestyle and behaviours became increasingly central to health promotion in the 1970s through programmes such as school educa-tion and *social marketing* campaigns around smoking, alcohol abuse, high fat foods and physical inactivity. Given the complex social and cultural circumstances associated with lifestyle, it is not surprising that many practitioners found that *health education* campaigns alone, a key strategy in the lifestyle approach, did not succeed in changing behaviour. The lifestyle approach does not necessarily view behaviour as an isolated action under the autonomous control of the individual, but recognizes how it is influenced and condi-tioned by a complex interplay of social, political and cultural factors. The lifestyle approach argued for a more comprehensive view to health promotion than simply health education about specific diseases. The *lifespan approach* also focuses on individual needs, but throughout our whole lives and like the lifestyle approach is based on providing appropriate interventions to promote healthy living (Hubley, Copeman and Woodall, 2013). Much of the health promo-tion work under the lifestyle approach continues to focus on the individual rather than on their context. Meredith Minkler (1989) argues that this is because many health promoters are embedded in both western and uniquely American value systems that place strong emphasis on the responsibility of the individual and the importance of autonomy and personal achievement.

The socio-environmental approach

The lifestyle approach presented health promoters with a complex interplay of social and cultural factors that only the most ambitious, long term and complicated of programmes could hope to achieve (Green and Kreuter, 2004). The critiques of the lifestyle approach gained momentum during the late 1970s and early 1980s when there was also a growing professional frustration with lifestyle models in health promotion because of the tendency to 'victim-blame', by assuming that individuals were responsible for their own actions. The lifestyle approach failed to recognize the structural issues, such as poverty, in which personal behaviours are embedded and which also indirectly but powerfully influence health. Inherent in the design of many of these programmes is a *power* struggle between professional and client and between communities and health promotion agencies who often identify the health issue(s) to be addressed. Social movements also challenged the notion of the medical and behavioural models to health by raising concerns for *social justice* and environmental sustainability. The critiques argued that health was primarily influenced by structural issues such as poverty, housing, over-population and lack of *community* control. A new, emancipatory discourse on health promotion began to form, one more concerned with social justice and ecological sustainability than with individual behaviour change. The socio-environmental approach viewed health as being influenced by high-risk social and environmental conditions and focused on how people could move to change them. The overall focus of health promotion shifted over time from thinking about whether the key interest is upon the individual (including biomedical and lifestyle aspects), community (including social supports and connections) or structural (including community resources, policy decisions and distribution of economic resources).

The ecological approach

The ecological approach of health promotion is based in part on an understanding of human ecology as the interaction of culture with environment. The approach encompasses culture and the biosphere, which ultimately is our living planet. Health is understood in its holistic sense, so the health of the individual is at the centre of the ecosystem and has body, mind and spiritual dimensions. The approach has system levels extending outwards from the individual representing the family, the community and its built environment and the wider society and natural environment, exemplified by culture and biosphere. The approach integrates the social sciences in its upper half (psychology, sociology, economics, politics and anthropology) with the natural sciences in its lower half (physics, chemistry, biology, engineering and ecology). Finally, the approach indicates that the 'health care' system is only one determinant of health, albeit one that at least in theory integrates the physical and social sciences. The approach should not be seen as static, but rather as a dynamic three-dimensional approach in which the various elements 'change' in shape and size according to their relative importance over time and in different communities. Moreover, the approach is not definitive and all encompassing, in particular, it fails to explicitly address equity and sustainability. The approach does, however, provide a useful way of depicting some of the major *determinants of health* and makes it clear that no single strategy and no effort focused on only one aspect of the determinants of health can be wholly successful. It implies multi-level, multi-faceted, multi-disciplinary approaches for a health promotion approach (Hancock, 1993).

Despite the modest evidence for the success of the 'lifestyle and behavioural' approach, it remains a popular option for health promotion practice. This approach offers the simple logic of behaviour change through education and motivational strategies. The approach allows practitioners to use established methodologies and activities such as social marketing, *information, education and communication* and *peer education*.

A major challenge in health promotion remains how best to apply the correct theory to the appropriate practice context. Health promotion programmes often cover a range of issues, target groups, settings and cultural contexts and use overlapping approaches in their design. Therefore when planning a programme the tendency is to choose a simple approach or strategy as the focus to the work. Government health agendas also typically promote healthy lifestyles and the use of interventions to change 'unhealthy' individual behaviours. This is because it has offered (falsely) easily quantifiable and achievable results within a short time frame (Gangolli, Duggal and Shukla, 2005) and financial incentives for savings in health care services, especially for people suffering from chronic diseases (Bernier, 2007).

Realistically, in practice, there is no one correct approach and the practitioner must be prepared to take the time to develop their capacity to operate at multiple theoretical levels with competing theories, models and approaches.

KEY TEXTS

- Naidoo, J. and Wills, J. (2009) *Foundations of Health Promotion.* 3rd edn (London: Bailliere and Tindall)
- Nutbeam, D., Harris, E. and Wise, M. (2010) *Theory in a Nutshell: A Practical Guide to Health Promotion Theories.* 3rd edn (Maidenhead: McGraw-Hill)
- Tones, K. and Tilford, S. (2001) *Health Education: Effectiveness, Efficiency and Equity.* 3rd edn (Cheltenham: Nelson Thornes)

b

behaviour change communication

SEE ALSO civil society; counselling and one-to-one communication; health literacy; information, education and communication

Behaviour change communication is an intervention to promote positive health behaviours that are appropriate to people's *settings* (UNDP, 2002).

A 'health behaviour' is any activity undertaken by an individual, regardless of actual or perceived health status, for the purpose of promoting, protecting or maintaining health, whether or not such behaviour is objectively effective towards that end. Almost every behaviour or activity by an individual has an impact on their health and it is therefore useful to distinguish between behaviours that are purposefully adopted to promote or protect health, and those which may be adopted regardless of the consequences to health (WHO, 1998). Providing people with information and teaching them how to behave does not necessarily lead to a desirable change in their behaviour. However, when there is a supportive environment plus an effective communication strategy, there is a greater chance of a desirable change in the behaviour of the target group.

Behaviour change communication has a close relation with information education and communication, *health education* and health communication. However, it is different from other instructional methods of communication because it is target specific and systematically considers the following in its design: the vulnerability/risk factor of the target group; the conflict and obstacles in the way to the desired change in behaviour; type of message and communication *media* that can best reach the target group and type of resources available and assessment of existing knowledge of the target group about the issue (UNDP, 2002).

The ideological foundation for a behaviour change communication approach is based on the assumption that before individuals and communities can change their behaviours, they must first understand basic facts about a particular health issue, adopt key attitudes, learn a set of skills and be given access to appropriate products and services. They must also perceive their environment as supporting their behaviour change and the maintenance of safe behaviours, as well as being supportive of seeking appropriate treatment for prevention, care and support, if necessary. This process has been identified as having a number of key steps centred around the provision and acceptance of new information and skills including pre-knowledge, becoming more knowledgeable, having a positive attitude towards the new knowledge, intending to take action to change their behaviour, practicing and advocating the behaviour (Corcoran, 2013).

Behaviour change communication has relied upon top-down, one-directional methods, such as the mass media, and this may have contributed to the causes for the gap between knowledge and practice (UNICEF, 2001). For example, in Vietnam 99% of people interviewed nationally were found to be aware of the link between iodine deficiency and goitre following a mass media campaign. However, supplementary iodized salt intake in some regions, such as the Mekong Delta, remained lower (68%) than the national average intake (77%) (National Iodine Deficiency Disorder Control Program, 2000). Other causes of this gap include a reliance on didactic styles of communication, inadequate audience segmentation, and inappropriate message content and poor materials development. This can be prevented by employing strategies that create a two-way communication between the recipient and a 'significant other' source of information, for example, a family member or health professional. A two-way communication creates a dialogue in which barriers to resolving health problems can be identified and actions to address the issue can be planned. To be effective, behaviour change communication must therefore use strategies that involve the development of a dialogue with the intended target group or individual including one-to-one communication, *self-help groups, health literacy* and interactive information and communication technologies.

KEY TEXTS
- Harnik, R. (2002) *Public Health Communication: Evidence for Behaviour Change* (New York: Routledge)

- Simons-Morton, B., McLeroy, K.C. and Wendel, M.L. (2011) *Behavior Theory in Health Promotion Practice and Research* (New York: Jones and Bartlett Learning)
- UNDP (2002) *Communication Behaviour Change Tools: Entertainment-Education*, Vol. 1 (New York: UNICEF), pp. 1–6

best practice

SEE evidence-based practice

bottom-up and top-down

SEE ALSO lay epidemiology; needs assessment; parallel-tracking

The way in which health concerns are to be addressed and are defined in a health promotion programme can take two distinct forms: bottom-up and top-down. A bottom-up approach encourages the *community* to identify its own problems and communicates these to those (above) who often have decision making authority (Laverack, 2004). In contrast, top-down describes programmes where problem identification comes from those in top structures 'down' to the community.

What should be remembered is that the terms top-down and bottom-up are ideal types of health promotion practice that are used to demonstrate important differences in relation to programme design (Laverack, 2004). They often have different agendas that create a bottom-up versus top-down 'tension'. The practitioner 'pushes-down' a pre-defined agenda onto the community through vertical programming. The community attempts to 'push-up' an agenda based on their immediate concerns that may not be the same as those identified by the practitioner. Top-down programmes would include almost all *health education* and multi-risk factor reduction interventions such as lifestyle and behaviour *approaches* that are the predominant style of health promotion programming. Bottom-up programmes are fewer in design and often exist as a part of larger scale top-down programme. To distinguish between a top-down and bottom-up programme design, it is useful to consider the following key questions:

1. **Does the programme have a fixed timeframe or a flexible timeframe?**

Top-down programmes have a fixed and specific timeframe, typically 1–3 years, to allow the funding agency to plan its technical inputs within expenditure cycles. In contrast, a longer timeframe is sometimes necessary to achieve bottom-up goals, typically 5–7 years. Requests for an extension of the timeframe of bottom-up programmes can be viewed by funding agencies as a failure to meet its objectives. To overcome this issue, the programme should have a more flexible timeframe. Some of the outcomes may be achieved within a relatively short timeframe; however, as this cannot always be guaranteed, an *evaluation* of the process (rather than solely the outcome) will provide evidence of the success of continuing bottom-up successes.

2. Is it the outside agent or the community who identifies the concerns to be addressed?

Both the outside agent and the community have concerns that they wish to address. The concerns of the outside agent are typically based on top-down procedures that employ forms of data collection such as epidemiological studies and systematic reviews. The concerns of communities are typically based on meeting their immediate needs or addressing local issues. Sometimes the concerns of the outside agent and the community are similar and can be reconciled in the design of the programme. More often, the concerns of the outside agent and the community are dissimilar, and a compromise has to be found.

3. Is it the outside agent or the community that has control over the management of the programme?

Top-down programmes are conventionally managed by an outside agent. The members of the community are expected to co-operate and contribute to the programme under the instruction of the management. Bottom-up approaches consciously involve the community in the management of the programme through skills training and by increasingly devolving responsibility for activities such as planning, report writing, budgeting and evaluation.

4. How is the programme evaluated?

If evaluation is concerned with targets and outcomes and is carried out by the outside agent or by independent 'experts', it is typically top-down. If evaluation is concerned with capacity building and processes that actively involves community participation, it is typically bottom-up.

The challenge to practitioners is how they can accommodate bottom-up approaches within the more dominant top-down styles of health promotion programming. This requires a fundamental change in the way we think about health promotion programming. Rather than viewing the issue as a bottom-up versus top-down tension, the process can be better viewed as a 'parallel track' running alongside the main 'programme track'. The tensions between the two styles of programming then occur at each stage of the programme cycle, making their resolution easier to achieve. 'Parallel-tracking' helps to move our thinking on theoretically from a simple bottom-up/top-down dichotomy and provides a systematic way in which to accommodate the two styles of programming (Laverack, 2007).

KEY TEXTS
- Laverack, G. (2007) *Health Promotion Practice: Building Empowered Communities* (Maidenhead: Open University Press)
- Laverack, G. and Labonte, R. (2000) 'A Planning Framework for the Accommodation of Community Empowerment Goals within Health Promotion Programming', *Health Policy and Planning*, 15 (3): pp. 255–262
- Baum, F. (2007) 'Cracking the Nut of Health Equity: Top Down and Bottom Up Pressure for Action on the Social Determinants of Health', *IUHPE Promotion and Education*, 14 (2): pp. 90–95

boycotts

SEE ALSO **health activism; information and communication technologies; lobbying**

A boycott is an act of voluntarily abstaining from using, buying or dealing with a person, organization or product as an expression of protest, usually for political reasons (Metoyer, 2007).

Boycotts are normally considered a one-time event to address a specific issue, although it may be for a longer period of time, or as part of an overall strategy. Boycotts not only use conventional tactics such as a civil protest but can also use electronic media such as mass e-mailing and virtual 'sit-ins' in an attempt to influence opinion (Metoyer, 2007). Consumer boycotts are focused on long-term change of buying habits and are usually part of a larger strategy aiming for the reform of consumer markets, or government commitment to the moral purchasing of products. Consumer boycotting was a tactic of activists in the 1960s and 1970s to try and punish corporations. By the 1990s, however, the trend was more towards developing standards and accrediting retail products that would be rewarded by consumers. Concerns have been raised that boycotting products manufactured through child labour, for example, may force children to turn to more dangerous sources of income. UNICEF has estimated that 50,000 children were dismissed from their garment industry jobs in Bangladesh following the introduction of the Child Labour Deterrence Act in the United States in the 1990s. Many children then resorted to jobs such as stone-crushing, street hustling and prostitution, jobs that are more hazardous and exploitative than garment production. The study suggests that some product boycotts can have long-term negative consequences that actually harm rather than help children employed in low-income jobs (UNICEF, 2001a).

The purpose of using boycotting in health promotion is at the heart of the role of the practitioner to promote informed choice and autonomous decision making. The role of the health promotion practitioner is as an enabler to support others to facilitate change in their lives through their own actions. Tactics such as consumer boycotting, in which the role of the practitioner is to guide interest groups on what is possible, can help others to increase control. Boycotts were a key strategy for the breastfeeding movement in an attempt to gain a greater influence over corporation consumer policy. Around the turn of the twentieth century, companies had begun marketing bovine milk products as infant food. By the 1950s, bottle-feeding was fashionable and considered to be superior to breastfeeding. In the 1960s, the milk formula industry embarked on an aggressive marketing campaign in the developing world. However, early breastfeeding advocates argued that formula was expensive for poor families and had negative health consequences for babies. Meanwhile, in industrialized countries, middle-class women argued that breastfeeding was an important aspect of mothering. Since then, an internationally organized breastfeeding movement has formed to challenge multinational corporations, to influence international policy and to educate and support breast-feeding women throughout the world. The breastfeeding movement gained momentum to organize a boycott of Nestlé products, a major manufacturer of infant milk formula, throughout the United States and this was soon emulated in Europe, Canada, New Zealand and Australia. The International Code of Marketing Infant Formula of 1981 stated that companies should accurately label their products, minimize advertising, avoid distributing free samples to mothers and maintain high quality standards. Because of corporate counter *lobbying*, the code was passed as a recommendation by the World Health Organization (WHO, which is more difficult to enforce) rather than as a regulation. In response, various grassroots organizations soon formed the International Baby Food Action Network (IBFAN) to promote the code and monitor the formula industry's compliance. In 1984, the Nestlé boycott was suspended after the company agreed to abide by the code. After numerous warnings, the boycott was resumed again in 1988 and was extended to other formula companies due to grievous code violations (Metoyer, 2007).

KEY TEXTS

- Friedman, M. (1999) *Consumer Boycotts: Effecting Change through the Marketplace and Media* (New York: Routledge)
- Laverack, G. (2013) *Health Activism: Foundations and Strategies* (London: Sage Publications), Chapter 8

C

civil society

SEE ALSO alliances, coalitions and partnerships; community; empowerment; health activism; networks

Civil society includes people in both their social and professional contexts who share a common set of interests or concerns, including the totality of voluntary civic and social organizations and institutions and which form the basis of a functioning society (Putnam, 1993).

The exact *definition* of civil society is debatable as, for example, the aforementioned interpretation of civil society does not include formal state or market activity, but it does include institutions that are opposed to the state and corporations. Civil society is important to health promotion because it stresses the need for a developed level of public and political participation and shares the core values of *empowerment* and emancipation.

Civil society is a much broader concept than that of a '*community*' as it refers to a diversity of spaces, actors and institutional forms, varying in their degree of formality, autonomy and *power*. Civil society works through people who create groups, organizations, communities and movements to address shared needs. Civil societies are populated by organizations such as registered charities, non-governmental organizations, community groups, women's organizations, faith-based organizations, trade unions, *self-help groups*, social movements and activist and *advocacy* groups (Laverack, 2007, p. 18).

The concept of civil society serves as an important point of entry for an analysis of many social, economic and political issues. The broad range of interests that make up civil society are often engaged in competition with one another and with formal state and market activities in order to increase their control over the influences in their lives. For example, large commercial and corporate lobbies have far more influence than ordinary citizens, *pressure groups*, movements or health promotion agencies. Companies contribute to society in many positive ways, but they can also put their interests ahead of the public interest and find political allies in trying to marginalize or counter the tactics used by others that are against their agenda. There are sophisticated public relations, market research and *lobbying* companies specializing in these types of counter tactics in support of, and often only within the financial reach of, corporations (Hager, 2009). Formal state organizations that pursue a tighter political and economic agenda have to reduce social structures, deregulate labour and financial markets and stimulate commerce and investment. For everyday living conditions, this means cutting pay and jobs, freezing benefits and welfare payments and reducing responsibility by transforming national health services into insurance-based health care systems, by privatizing medical care and by promoting a model of health as individualized (Navarro, 2009). Civil society is given little opportunity to express their discontent through traditional channels such as local and national voting. Instead this leaves civil society with only one option: to engage in action that goes beyond what is conventional or routine through activism (Laverack, 2013).

This raises the question of the role of the state in support of civil society. Two fundamentally different positions on this role are evident: libertarian and communitarian. The libertarian position sees the development of civil society as a means of 'rolling back the state'. The state is seen to interfere in the development of civil society by restricting the freedom of individuals. By contrast communitarians see a central role of the state as advancing the development of civil society through the provision of state-funded structures to support and nurture it. There is not a simple solution, especially in fiscal climates that encourage individualism and the libertarian approach over a broader structural and community approach. However, neither is it an either or situation. Historically, what has defined a successful and contemporary practice has been the willingness of the state to work with others to address the causes of social injustice and health inequities in civil society (Baum, 1997).

Civil society has a broad range of intentions, both positive and negative, and there is therefore an element of 'uncivil society' that acts as a counterweight to an overly optimistic vision of what civil society is or can achieve. Ironically, while many policy makers are concerned with the challenge of building civil society in transitional and developing countries, there is a feeling in many industrialized countries that civil society has been degraded and has become less a feature of everyday life. The concept of civil society has therefore been criticized as a 'feel-good' factor that does not always account for conservative or repressive forces in the political arena (Lewis, 2003).

KEY TEXTS
- Eberly, D. (2008) *The Rise of Global Civil Society: Building Communities and Nations from the Bottom Up* (New York: Encounter books)
- Edwards, M. (2009) *Civil Society.* 2nd edn (Oxford: Polity Press)
- Edwards, M. (2011) *The Oxford Handbook of Civil Society* (Oxford: Oxford University Press)

community

SEE ALSO **civil society; community-based intervention; information and communication technologies; community capacity; empowerment**

It is important to think beyond the customary view of a community as a place where people live, for example, a neighbourhood, because these are often just an aggregate of non-connected people. Communities have both a social and a geographic characteristic and consist of heterogeneous individuals with dynamic relations that sometimes organize into groups to take action towards achieving shared goals (Laverack, 2004).

As a working 'rule of thumb' a community will have the following characteristics:

1. a spatial dimension, that is, a place or locale;
2. non-spatial dimensions that involve people who otherwise make up heterogeneous and disparate groups;
3. social interactions that are dynamic and bind people into relationships and
4. the identification of shared needs and concerns (Laverack, 2004, p. 46).

Within the geographic dimensions of 'community', multiple non-spatial communities exist and individuals may belong to several different 'interest' groups at the same time. Interest groups exist as a legitimate means by which individuals can find a 'voice' and are able to participate to pursue their interests and concerns. Interest groups can be organized around a variety of social activities or can address a local and shared concern, for example, poor access to public transport. The diversity of individuals and groups within a community can create problems with regard to the selection of representation by its members (Zakus and Lysack, 1998). Practitioners try to work with the 'legitimate' representatives of a community and to avoid the establishment of a dominant minority that can dictate community issues based only on their own concerns and not on those of the majority. Practitioners need to carefully consider if the representatives of a community are, in fact, supported by its members and that they are not simply acting out of self-interest and self-gain.

Goodman *et al.* (1998) argue that a sense of community can be strengthened through a connection with or an understanding of its history. This is made up of events, people and experiences involving previous economic, political and socio-cultural contexts. Knowledge of the historical context of the community can help identify potential barriers such as experiences of conflict or feelings of helplessness and provide a better chance of affecting change than those that do not have access to this information.

With the advent of online communities, new types of computerized tools have been developed to aid user participation. *Information and communication technology* has removed the physical barriers to communication, for example, people are able to participate online in discussions that are classified by topic, each with many conversational threads from across the globe. Online communities, like traditional forms of community, consist of a diverse group of people who participate in virtual spaces with little social context and member identity. Social media can encourage communication by enabling participants to find others with whom they only share interests and by providing a means to contact them. This facilitates social interactions in online communities and promotes communication by creating chat spaces that allows the participants to perceive the number of people present and the level of their activity, just as they would in a room in the offline world. The internet has helped to promote 'global communities' and 'digital cities' by building arenas in which people can interact, share knowledge, experience and mutual interests. However, online activity is still limited to those who are computer literate and have access to a computer and the internet and this can exclude many people (Nomura and Ishida, 2003).

KEY TEXTS
- Block, P. (2009) *Community: The Structure to Belonging* (San Francisco, CA: Berrett-Koehler Publishers)
- Delanty, G. (2003) *Community* (New York: Routledge)
- Zakus, J.D.L. and Lysack, C.L. (1998) 'Revisiting Community Participation', *Health Policy and Planning*, 13 (1): pp. 1–12

community-based intervention

SEE ALSO civil society; community; community capacity building; empowerment; lay epidemiology

Community-based interventions are designed to work with people to address their needs. They can help practitioners to better engage with, organize and mobilize communities. They can also help practitioners to appreciate the role that they have in facilitating community participation, action and *empowerment* in their everyday work (Laverack, 2007).

As communities build their level of social and organizational interaction, they become more concerned about, and ready to address, the broader determinants on the lives of their members. The key point is that at some stage communities are no longer just passive participants but will take an active role in identifying and resolving their own concerns to address the underlying causes of their *powerlessness* and in turn will become engaged in politically orientated activities.

While there is not a hierarchy or linear progression of community-based interventions, in practice they are often implemented as a dynamic process. The main community-based interventions used in health promotion are readiness, participation, engagement, organization, development, capacity building, action and empowerment. Each of these is next discussed in relation to one another and in terms of how they are used in health promotion.

Community readiness is a state of *community* preparedness to engage in a partnership with an outside agent to implement a health promotion programme. To reach this state, communities move through a series of stages to develop and implement effective programmes. The measure of preparedness is not the level of ease or difficulty with which the changes from one stage to another are made but the readiness or un-readiness of a community to accept the change (Plested, Edwards and Jumper-Thurman, 2003). Community readiness implies a willingness to engage with an intervention but not a previous history of participation between the members of the community. Community readiness is typically measured using questionnaires and interviews to obtain information from people by an outside agency.

Community participation allows people to address a broad range of common needs by sharing their ideas and experiences (Rifkin, 1990). In practice, participation is more likely to be the representation of the majority by a few, for example, through an elected individual to sit on an advisory committee. However, participation can become empty and frustrating for those whose involvement is passive and that in effect allows those in authority to claim that all sides were considered while only a few benefit.

Community engagement takes participation a step further by including people in identifying problem-solving solutions to issues that affect their lives. There are many models of community engagement, for example, the consultation–public participation approach, the asset-based-social economy approach, the community-democracy approach and the community-organizing approach (Hashagen, 2002). Community engagement is a collaborative process, often between an outside agency and the community and includes the following steps: listening and communication; participation; *needs assessment* and working together in partnerships.

From this point forward, community-based intervention is concerned with people taking actions by which to resolve the issues that they have identified. Community-based intervention progresses from being participatory to becoming more systematic and action orientated. A community that is action orientated is better able to organize and mobilize itself towards addressing shared goals.

Community organization allows people to take a role in shared decision making and problem solving that is based on their own self-determination (Braithwaite, Bianchi and Taylor, 1994). Historically, the concept of organizing communities was developed, from the programme planner's point of view, to explain a way that people could decrease disease and increase their quality of life. The root of community organization is based on the work of Saul Alinsky (1972) whose underlying philosophy was that the people should be in control of their own lives. Organization and development, linked to a collective struggle, is seen by those working with communities as a legitimate approach to improve the health and lives of others.

Community development takes health promoters a step further by providing a means by which outside agencies can enable communities to improve their lives. This is through activities and interventions such as education, skills training and technical support. Community development is often linked to the distribution of resources and to economic, infrastructural and political opportunities as well as to social development (Labonte, 1998). Community development is often an aspect of state policy and, therefore, remains enmeshed within the dominance of top-down programmes (Petersen, 1994). For example, community development has been used in neighbourhood-based projects that are set up with government support, including an appointed community worker, to address issues of local concern (Jones and Sidell, 1997). Community-based rehabilitation (CBR) is a strategy within general community development for the rehabilitation, equalization of opportunities, poverty reduction and social inclusion of people with disabilities. CBR programmes are mostly in resource-poor areas and are usually implemented through the combined efforts of people with disabilities, their families, community workers, health professionals and communities. It includes work to promote social inclusion, empowerment, as well as access to education, to decent work opportunities, and to preventive, rehabilitative and curative health services (ILO, UNESCO and WHO, 2004).

Community capacity was developed more recently (Goodman *et al.*, 1998) than community development to provide a systematic approach to build the assets and attributes of a community within the design of a programme. This has been possible because of the advances made in interpreting this complex concept, for example, the 'domains' of community capacity are areas of influence that allow communities to better organize and mobilize themselves towards social and political change.

Although capacity builds the assets and attributes of people, community action is the resolution of their concerns to take specific actions to achieve self-identified goals. Communities have ownership of the issues that concern them (Boutilier, 1993) and control who identifies the issues to be addressed in a programme. Together, community action and community control are the basis for self-determination that gives people the purpose and direction to improve their lives. Community action often begins when people come together to address local concerns for short-term periods of time. These groups can form into NIMBY's (Not In My Back Yard) directed at local issues, for example, the development of a new road that would spoil the natural beauty of the environment. To achieve their actions, communities must possess the necessary resources and the preparedness to engage with outside agencies. At this point, communities have reached a state of self-determination and are focussed on achieving goals through their own actions.

The key difference between community empowerment and the other community-based interventions is the sense of struggle and liberation that is bound in the process of gaining *power*. Community empowerment builds from the individual to the group to a wider collective and embodies the intention to bring about social and political change. The overlap between community-based interventions often lies in how and why people interact. The similarity lies in the process that people follow. The difference lies in the intended purpose or outcome. The purpose may initially be as simple as the participation of people. Later this becomes more concerned with building the *competencies* and capacities of people directed towards specific goals and actions. But only when these goals are achieved through long-lasting social and political change do communities really begin to empower themselves.

KEY TEXTS
- CDC/ATSDR. Committee on Community Engagement (1997) *Principles of Community Engagement* (Atlanta: GA), pp. 62–63

- Laverack, G. (2007) *Health Promotion Practice: Building Empowered Communities* (Maidenhead: Open University Press), Chapter 2
- Plested, B., Edwards, R. and Jumper-Thurman, P. (2003) *Community Readiness – The Key to Successful Change* (The Tri-ethnic Center for Prevention Research, Sage Hall. Fort Collins, CO: Colorado State University)

community capacity building

SEE ALSO **alliances, partnerships and coalitions; civil society; community; empowerment; evaluation**

Community capacity building is the increase in *community* groups' abilities to define, assess, analyse and act on health (or any other) concerns of importance to their members (Labonte and Laverack, 2001a, p. 114). Generally, it is viewed as a process that increases the assets and attributes that a community is able to draw upon (Goodman *et al.*, 1998).

Community capacity building is not specific to a particular locality, nor of the individuals or groups within it, but of the inter-actions between both. Interest in capacity building as a strategy for sustainable skills, resources and commitments in various *settings* has developed because of the requirement to prolong project gains (Gibbon, Labonte and Laverack, 2002). For a health promotion organization or health promoter, the task is not to create a new programme called 'capacity building'; rather, the task is to examine how its practice can support the development of capacity building. Capacity building becomes the process by which the end result of increasing community control and programme sustainability can be achieved through, for example, increasing knowledge and developing skills and *competencies*.

Community *empowerment* and capacity building overlap closely as forms of social organization and social mobilization that seek to address the inequalities in peoples' lives (Laverack, 2007). Community capacity building is often the means by which the outcome of increased community empowerment can be achieved. However, the process of both community capacity building and empowerment are achieved through systematically building knowledge, skills and competencies at an individual and collective level.

While there is a broad body of literature with regard to the *definition* and assessment of community capacity, the discussion offers little with regard to how to make this concept operational in a health promotion programme context. However, in recent years, for example, the concept of community capacity has been 'unpacked' into the organizational areas of influence that significantly contribute to its development (Labonte and Laverack, 2001b). The 'capacity domains' represent those aspects of the process of community capacity that allow individuals and groups to better organize and mobilize themselves towards gaining greater control of their lives. The 'capacity domains' provide a pre-determined focus to build community capacity to: improve stakeholder participation; develop local *leadership*; build organizational structures; increase problem assessment capacities; enhance stakeholder ability to 'ask why'; improve resource mobilization; strengthen links to other organizations and people; create an equitable relationship with outside agents and increase stakeholder control over programme management (Laverack, 2001). The existence of each of these domains is indicative of a robust and capable community, one that has strong organizational and social abilities (Laverack, 2004).

In practice, health promotion is implemented as a set of activities within the context of an intervention, a project or a programme. The 'programme' is conventionally managed and monitored by, for example, a health promotion practitioner and commonly includes a period of identification, design, implementation, management and *evaluation*. The basic question planners and practitioners need to ask themselves is: How has the health promotion programme helped to increase community capacity? *Approaches* to build community capacity are intended to be an empowering experience for communities and therefore involve the use of participatory 'tools' to enable people to better organize themselves and to strategically plan for actions to resolve their circumstances, to evaluate and ideally to visually represent the outcomes (Laverack, 2007). A period of observation and discussion is important to first adapt the approach to the social and cultural requirements of the participants. For example, the use of a working definition of community capacity building can provide all participants with a more mutual understanding of the concept in which they are involved and towards which they are expected to contribute. Measurement is by itself insufficient to build capacity as this information must also be transformed into actions. This is achieved through strategic planning for positive changes to achieve improvements at an individual and a community level. The participants usually develop a detailed strategy based on identifying specific activities; sequencing activities into the correct order to make an improvement; setting a realistic time frame including any targets and assigning individual responsibilities to complete each activity within the programme time frame. The participants will also have to assess the resources that are necessary and available to improve their present situation.

The early experiences of the evaluation of community capacity used qualitative information to provide 'thick' descriptive accounts based on the experiences of the participants that produced a large quantity of data such as transcribed interviews. This type of data was difficult and time consuming for practitioners to interpret. The lessons learnt from these experiences have provided the basis for the subsequent development of approaches that are intended to be an empowering experience for communities. It enables people to participate, to better organize themselves and to critically reflect on their individual and collective circumstances. More importantly, it enables people to strategically plan for actions to resolve their circumstances, to measure and to visually represent this process as outcomes that are conducive to health promotion programming. In particular, visual representation of the findings produces a graphic image of the personal experiences of the participants in a format that is concise and measurable. The visualization of such a complex concept presents an attractive option to practitioners who may wish to make a representation of the analysis, over a specific time frame, and in a way that can be understood by all the programme stakeholders, including the community members.

KEY TEXTS

- Goodman, R.M. *et al.* (1998) 'Identifying and Defining the Dimensions of Community Capacity to Provide a Basis for Measurement', *Health Education & Behavior*, 25 (3): pp. 258–278
- Labonte, R. and Laverack, G. (2001a) 'Capacity Building in Health Promotion, Part 1: For Whom? And for What Purpose?' *Critical Public Health*, 11 (2): pp. 111–127

- Labonte, R. and Laverack, G. (2001b) 'Capacity Building in Health Promotion, Part 2: Whose Use? And with What Measure?' *Critical Public Health*, 11 (2): pp. 129–138

competencies

SEE ALSO **advocacy; definition; leadership; power**

Competencies are a combination of attributes including knowledge, skills and values that enable an individual to perform a set of tasks to an appropriate standard for the practice of health promotion (Dempsey, Battel-Kirk and Barry, 2011).

Health promotion practitioners are expected to display a specialization of knowledge, technical competence, social responsibility and service to their clients. Their level of professionalism is attained through education, training, professional codes of practice and core competencies. Core competencies for health promotion include not only practical knowledge and skills but also the values and principles that shape the professional practice. Core competencies also provide a set of standards by which the workforce can determine what a 'professional' practice is and can be used to set parameters for staff development, recruitment and performance standards (Laverack, 2007).

For some practitioners, health promotion is only a small part of their daily work, for example, a nurse who undertakes a mix of clinical practice and *health education*. Different professional groups have developed their own sets of generic competencies to provide the minimum entry level of competence to meet a professional standard, for example, to deliver essential nursing services. For practitioners who are not solely involved in health promotion, it is their responsibility to select which specialist competencies they feel are most relevant to their work.

The development of a Europe-wide system of competency-based standards in health promotion has aimed to provide the basis for building a competent and effective health promotion workforce. The CompHP Project, for example, aimed to develop competency-based standards and an accreditation system for health promotion practice, education and training that positively impacts on workforce capacity to deliver health improvement. The project worked through existing health promotion *networks* across Europe to develop and test the implementation of a sustainable competency-based system in countries with varying levels of infrastructure development. The purpose was to develop core competencies that can be adapted within agreed parameters at national levels. The CompHP Project identified that ethical values, including a belief in equity and *social justice*, and health promotion knowledge, underpin the competencies framework. The project identified a further nine domains that related to a specific area of work in health promotion and a number of associated competencies for each area. The nine domains are as follows: enable change; advocate for health; mediate through partnership; communication; *leadership*; assessment; planning; implementation and *evaluation* and research. A combined application of all these domains constituted a professional competencies framework for health promotion.

An international consensus meeting to identify core competencies, jointly organized by the International Union for Health Promotion and Education (IUHPE), the Society for Public Health Education (SOPHE) and the US Centers for Disease Control (CDC), with participation from international leaders in the field, took place at the National University of Ireland, Galway, in June 2008. The purpose of the meeting was to strengthen global exchange, collaboration and common *approaches* to capacity building and workforce development in health promotion. The consensus statement of the meeting outlines core values and principles, a common *definition* and eight domains of core competency that are required to engage in effective health promotion practice. The core domains of competency agreed to at the meeting are catalyzing change, leadership, assessment, planning, implementation, evaluation, *advocacy* and partnerships (Barry *et al.*, 2009).

A further comparative list of core competencies is given below, and although not exhaustive, it does provide examples of what is required to allow health promotion practitioners to grow and develop as professionals.

1. **Programme design, management, implementation and evaluation.**
The ability to plan effective health promotion programmes, including the management of resources and personnel. This involves an understanding of programme cycles, budgeting, the planning and evaluation of bottom-up approaches in top-down programming.

2. The planning and delivery of effective communication strategies.

Communication strategies are an integral part of many health promotion programmes to increase knowledge levels and to raise awareness. A high level of competence is needed for the development of programmes that target individuals, groups and communities including one-to-one communication, the design of print materials and the use of the mass media.

3. Facilitating skills.

Training, for example, for skills development, usually within a workshop setting, is a key part of many health promotion programmes. Good facilitation skills are essential for health promoters and are an important part of programme design.

4. Research skills.

Health promotion programme design and evaluation is based on sound research including the use of participatory techniques, qualitative and quantitative methods and systematic reviews.

5. Community capacity building skills.

Community empowerment is central to health promotion. This is a process of capacity building and health promoters must be competent in a range of strategies that they can use to help individuals, groups and communities to gain more *power*.

6. Ability to influence policy and practice.

Health promoters have the opportunity to influence policy and practice in their everyday work, for example, through technical advisory groups and through helping communities to mobilize and organize themselves towards gaining power. Health promoters must develop competence in the use of strategies to influence policy, developing partnerships and sound working relationships (Laverack, 2007).

KEY TEXTS

- Barry, M. *et al.* (2009) 'The Galway Conference Statement: International Collaboration on the Development of Core Competencies for Health Promotion and Health Education', *Global Health Promotion*, 16 (2): pp. 5–11

- Dempsey, C., Battel-Kirk, B. and Barry, M. (2011) *The CompHP Core Competencies Framework for Health Promotion Handbook* (Executive Agency for Health and Consumers, Paris: IUHPE)
- Holmes, L. (2008) *Basics of Public Health Core Competencies* (Boston, MA: Jones and Bartlett Learning)
- Perez, M. and Luquis, R. (2008) *Cultural Competence in Health Education and Health Promotion* (San Francisco, CA: Jossey-Bass)

conflict resolution

SEE ALSO **counselling and one-to-one communication; empowerment; leadership; power**

Conflict resolution are the methods and processes involved in facilitating the peaceful ending of conflict by individuals or group members by actively communicating information about their conflicting motives or ideologies to others and by engaging in collective negotiation (Forsyth, 2009).

Conflict can be a negative ingredient of the health promotion interventions primarily by taking attention away from important issues, by dividing *community* groups and by undermining individuals' power-from-within. However, if managed correctly it can also be a positive ingredient. Dealing with conflict in a positive way can resolve disputes, help to release emotions and anxieties and make people address sensitive issues while at the same time improving co-operation and communication. The beginnings of conflict are often caused by poor communication between individual stakeholders and between interest groups, weak local *leadership*, internal struggles to gain access to limited resources, struggles between the powerless and those seen to hold the *power* and the uncertainty of practitioners about their role in resolving conflict (Laverack, 2009).

In conflict situations, those with the power over tend to try to dominate, to use pressure tactics and to offer few concessions, and this can make it difficult to reach a negotiated agreement that is satisfactory to all parties. Those who are in a powerless position become alienated and either resist by increasing their own power base and using tactics of disobedience and activism or to induce those with power to use it more benevolently and to be sympathetic of the inequality of those with less power (Coleman, 2000). The health promotion practitioner can play an important role in resolving conflict by simply assessing the situation, being a good listener and inviting stakeholder participation to clarify areas of conflict. An example of resolving cross-cultural differences is the 'Aik Saath Project', which was started to address inter-ethnic tension and outbreaks of conflict between the Sikh and Muslim youth in Slough, the United Kingdom. The role of locally recruited and trained facilitators in conflict resolution played a major role in reducing tensions, such as the number of playground fights between Sikhs and Muslims, and in building a working relationship with street gangs. The Project also used local conflict resolution groups and worked in schools to identify and address the key issues causing the tensions. The conflict resolution groups were made up of students from each year and provided an important entry point into the school and into the issues facing youth on inter-ethnic conflict. The groups provided a bridge between the practitioners and their clients, the youth, and so it was important to carefully manage their development. The Project found that in order to develop a conflict resolution group it was necessary to: carefully select the targeted youth; work with existing community-based organizations in contact with the youth; invest in young people to act as facilitators and provide them with outreach resources; have mechanisms to value their input; engage with key public sector agencies and have a realistic timeframe to achieve your aims (renewal.net, 2008).

Conflict resolution does not have to be a specialist area of work especially when the issue of disagreement is not complicated and can be resolved by a simple clarification and discussion of the main concerns. There are a number of different theories and models for conflict resolution, notably negotiation, mediation, diplomacy and creative peacemaking. The dual concern model, for example, involves all stakeholders in equal decision making about concerns for themselves and for others (Forsyth, 2009). However, conflict resolution can be quite simply facilitated by the practitioner using participatory *approaches* to first map the main questions and issues held between the different stakeholders involved and then by developing strategies to discuss and address each concern.

KEY TEXTS

- Coleman, P.T. (2000) 'Power and Conflict' in M. Deutsch and P.T. Coleman (eds), *The Handbook of Conflict Resolution: Theory and Practice* (San Francisco, CA: Jossey-Bass)
- Dana, D. (2000) *Conflict Resolution* (London: McGraw-Hill)
- Forsyth, D.R. (2009) *Group Dynamics*. 5th edn (Singapore: Cengage Learning)

counselling and one-to-one communication

SEE ALSO behaviour change communication; information, education and communication; moral suasion; patient empowerment; power; self-help

Counselling refers to any form of interaction where someone seeks to explore, understand or resolve a problem or a troubling personal aspect of their life. Counselling occurs broadly when a person consults someone else with regard to a problem, conflict or dilemma that is preventing them from living their lives in a way that they would wish to do so (McLeod and McLeod, 2011, p. 1).

Counselling emerged as a profession in the twentieth century, splitting from therapeutic *approaches* and developing its own professional field, although still retaining much in common with therapy. The field developed quickly with the formation of many different modalities including biblical, marriage, mental health, emotional, school and grief counselling. Essentially, counselling can involve people working in any kind of helping, managing or in a facilitative role such as social work, health professionals and teachers. Counsellors help clients explore and understand their worlds and so discover better ways of thinking and living. This can be done for one person or a group (typically couples and families) and may be delivered through a number of methods such as one-to-one communication, group work (Dryden and Feltham, 1993) interpersonal communication, interviewing and shared decision making. However, it is important to emphasize that the choice of the communication style in counselling is usually at the discretion of the practitioner, who decides, based on the circumstances and the type of client, what is most acceptable.

A common factor in most counselling situations is that the client is emotionally distressed or otherwise in a negative state of mind about something and there is an ongoing debate about the difference between counselling and therapy. While the boundaries are not always clear, therapy can be used in a more clinical context while counselling tends to have a more social focus. A critical variable in the style of counselling used is the extent to which the solution to problems is provided by the counsellor or by the client. This leads to two very different roles for the counsellor: problem solver or facilitator (Dryden and Feltham, 1993).

One-to-one communication is individually focussed on a one (the agent/practitioner) to-one (the client) basis, for example, a doctor talking to a patient. One-to-one communication is important in counselling because this allows a dialogue to develop between the client and the practitioner. The dialogue is often based on a sharing of knowledge and experiences in a two-way communication that is necessary to help individuals to better retain information, to clarify personal issues and to develop skills. An example of using one-to-one communication in a counselling situation is helping someone understand a sensitive issue such as the result of a medical test (Hubley, Copeman and Woodall, 2013).

Language also exerts considerable force in our world constructions and this applies to our professional as well as our social worlds (Seidman and Wagner, 1992). In counselling, the advantage is often held by the one with the control, usually the practitioner, and the language that they choose to use can either strengthen or weaken the professional relationship. Technical terms are a part of the everyday language of practitioners, for example, medical diagnostic vocabulary, and have evolved as knowledge and skills develop within a profession's subculture (other subcultures include ethnic groups, social class and sexuality). However, the use of specialist language is often confusing to both lay people and practitioners not part of the professional subculture. This can contribute to their sense of *powerlessness* by showing a lack of access to knowledge and the 'expert' *power* of the other person using the language. Scrambler (1987) provides an example of a consultation between a health practitioner and a pregnant woman. The practitioner began the discussion using 'lay' terms to describe the complications associated with her condition but quickly switched to a technical-rational language when her advice was challenged by the pregnant woman. The woman was then coerced into complying with the practitioner because she suddenly felt uncertain and lacking in knowledge. The pregnant woman had been disempowered by the practitioner who said that she was unaware of the switch to a technical, power-over use of language. While it may sometimes be necessary to use specific technical terms, it is more empowering when using language and terminology that is understood by the receivers. This reduces any confusion, alienation or mystification on behalf of the receiver by the communicator. It is important for practitioners to understand the influence of their language and to be sensitive to the position and perceptions of others. Such awareness is termed as a 'reflexive practice' in which practitioners are critical about the way they use their knowledge and power to have influence over others.

To improve counselling, the practitioner can follow a simple procedure of listening, giving advice and obtaining and providing feedback to their clients. Listening is an active process focussing on what the individual is saying and if necessary helping the speaker to express his/her feelings or to give an opinion on an issue. When giving advice, the practitioner is exerting his/her expert and legitimate power to persuade the client into actually accepting a subservient role relationship. The relationship grants the practitioner the right to prescribe advice, while the client accepts an obligation to comply with the advice. This is sometimes a necessary communication style when, for example, giving a precise instruction such as the self-treatment of a wound by the patient to ensure their compliance. Obtaining and giving feedback enables the practitioner to clarify what the client wants and that they have understood previous communication or retained skills. This may mean obtaining feedback based on specific information using closed questions that require short factual (yes/no) answers or based on an open form of questioning to provide fuller answers. Giving feedback is important for the achievement of effective one-to-one communication and in particular positive feedback that reinforces the strengths of the client's knowledge level. The client is encouraged to share his/her concerns, feelings and opinions but the discussion is directed by the practitioner. To facilitate this process, the practitioner can use 'people-centred' approaches such as the patient-centred clinical method (Stewart, Brown and Weston, 2003) that applies the principles of *empowerment* in a practitioner–patient relationship.

KEY TEXTS

- Aldridge, S. and Rigby, S. (2001) *Counselling Skills in Context* (London: Hodder and Stoughton)
- Corcoran, N. (eds) (2013) *Communicating Health: Strategies for Health Promotion.* 2nd edn (London: Sage Publications)
- Hubley, J., Copeman, J. and Woodall, J. (2013) *Practical Health Promotion.* 2nd edn (Cambridge, UK: Polity Press)
- McLeod, J. and Mcleod, J. (2011) *A Practical Guide for Counsellors and Helping Professionals* (Maidenhead: Open University Press)

critical consciousness

SEE ALSO **empowerment; health literacy; photo-voice; power**

Critical consciousness can be described as '...the ability to reflect on the assumptions underlying our and others' ideas and actions and to contemplate alternative ways of living' (Goodman *et al.*, 1998, p. 272).

Communities cannot intentionally empower themselves without having an understanding of the underlying causes of their *power-lessness.* This may occur from within the *community* 'organically' or as an intervention driven by an outside agent as a process of discussion, reflection and action. This process is called 'critical consciousness' or 'conscientization' and involves emancipation through learning using, for example, 'empowerment education' as developed by the educationalist Paulo Freire (1973) from literacy programmes in Brazil. To Paulo Freire, the central premise was that education is not neutral but is influenced by the context of one's life. The purpose of education is liberation and emancipation in which people become the subjects of their own learning involving critical reflection and analysis of their personal circumstances (Wallerstein and Bernstein, 1988). To achieve this, Freire proposed a group dialogue approach to share ideas and experiences and to promote critical thinking by posing problems to allow people to uncover the root causes of their powerlessness. Once critically aware, people can then plan more effective actions to change their circumstances, a defining prerequisite in the process of *empowerment.* Paulo Freire showed that working to raise the critical consciousness of people with poor basic literacy skills can lead to outcomes that are closely aligned with empowerment (Nutbeam, 2000). The approach does involve a considerable commitment to be able to gradually understand the causes of powerlessness and to develop realistic actions to begin to resolve the structural conditions that created them in the first place. An example of how being critically conscious can influence health outcomes is provided through the use of '*photo-voice*' or 'photo-novella'. This is a 'tool' that enables people to identify, represent and enhance their lives through a specific photographic technique. It uses the immediacy of the visual image and accompanying stories to furnish evidence and to promote an effective, participatory means of sharing experiences to address people's powerlessness (Wang, Tao and Carvano, 1998).

KEY TEXTS
- Freire, P. (2005) *Education for Critical Consciousness* (New York: Continuum Press)
- Laverack, G. (2004) *Health Promotion Practice: Power and Empowerment* (London: Sage Publications), Chapter 7
- Hubley, J., Copeman, J. and Woodall, J. (2013) *Practical Health Promotion*. 2nd edn (Cambridge, UK: Polity Press)

d

declarations and statements

SEE ALSO approaches; definition; evidence-based practice;
public health; theory and models

For many years the WHO has provided the global direction and
leadership that has helped to shape the way we view health promotion. This has been marked by key international declarations and
statements that have helped to map, define and legitimize new
approaches to health promotion theory and practice. The WHO has
had a significant role in orchestrating these milestones through
its international convening powers, even though as an organization its role and influence in health promotion has diminished
in recent years because of global financial constraints (Laverack,
2012a).

The most notable WHO charters and statements have been the
1986 Ottawa Charter; the 1988 Adelaide Conference Statement; the
1991 Sundsvall Conference Statement; the 1997 Jakarta Conference
Statement; the 2000 Mexico Global Conference statement; the 2005
Bangkok Charter for Health Promotion in a Globalized World and
the 2009 global conference on health promotion. An interpretation
of each of these is given below.

The 1986 Ottawa Charter (WHO, 1986) for Health Promotion
was the first international conference and was primarily a response
to growing expectations for a new *public health* movement.

The Ottawa Charter 1986
Health promotion is the process of enabling people to increase
control over, and to improve, their health. To reach a state of
complete physical, mental and social wellbeing, an individual or a
group must be able to identify and to realize aspirations, to satisfy
needs and to change or cope with the environment. Health promotion is not just the responsibility of the health sector, but goes
beyond healthy lifestyles to wellbeing (WHO, 1986).

Discussions at the conference focussed on the needs of people in industrialized countries and built on progress made by an earlier declaration on *primary health care* in Alma Alta (WHO, 1978). The conference identified a number of prerequisites or fundamental conditions and resources that are crucial for the improvement of health, peace, shelter, education, food, income, a stable eco-system, sustainable resources, *social justice* and equity. The Charter expanded the outcomes for health promotion beyond the absence of disease or the adoption of healthy lifestyles. The Charter defined five health promotion action areas for achieving better health: (1) *building healthy public policy*; (2) creating supportive environments; (3) strengthening *community action*; (4) developing personal skills and (5) re-orienting health services. It also described three impor-tant roles for health promoters: *advocating*, enabling and mediating and became the founding document of the 'new' health promotion movement.

The 1988 Adelaide Conference Statement (WHO, 1988) addressed the first of the five action areas from the Ottawa Charter (WHO, 1986): building healthy public policy. The conference statement stated that 'health is both a fundamental human right and a sound social investment'. It went on to state that '... inequal-ities in health are rooted in inequalities in society. Closing the health gap would require public policy that improved access to health enhancing goods and services and created supportive environments.'

The 1991 Sundsvall Conference Statement (WHO, 1991) was the first WHO health promotion conference to have a global perspec-tive. This conference addressed the second of the five action areas for health promotion from the Ottawa Charter (WHO, 1986), creating supportive environments. This concept encompasses both the physical and social aspects of where people live, work and play. The conference highlighted four important aspects of supportive environments: (1) traditional values and beliefs, customs, social proc-esses and rituals that provide a sense of belonging, coherence and purpose; (2) governmental commitment to human rights, social justice, peace and democracy; (3) re-channelling economic resources into the achievement of 'health for all' and away from the arms race and (4) the important role of women in creating supportive environ-ments, and the need to stop their exploitation.

The 1997 Jakarta Conference Statement (WHO, 1997) endorsed health as a basic human right, affirmed the five action areas of the Ottawa Charter and proposed (somewhat controversially) that new partnerships, especially with the private sector, was important to the success of health promotion. The Conference Declaration also affirmed that there is clear evidence that:

- Comprehensive approaches to health development are the most effective.
- '*Settings*' (such as families, neighbourhoods and communities) for health offer practical opportunities for the implementation of comprehensive strategies.
- Participation by all people is essential to sustain efforts.
- *Health literacy* fosters participation.
- Access to education and information is essential to achieving effective participation and the *empowerment* of people and communities.

The 2000 Mexico Global Conference for Health Promotion (WHO, 2000) sought to demonstrate how health promotion strategies add value to the effectiveness of health and development policies, programmes and projects, particularly those that aim to improve the health and quality of life of people living in adverse circumstances. The Conference Statement recognized that health is not only an outcome of, but also an important input into, economic development and equity. It also declared that health promotion and social development 'is a central duty and responsibility of governments', and that 'health promotion must be a fundamental component of public policies and programmes in all countries in the pursuit of equity and better health for all.' The Conference challenged health promotion to pay closer attention to global phenomena, such as the re-appearance and broader spread of the HIV/AIDS pandemic in Africa and growing global disparities in wealth and health.

The 2005 Bangkok Charter for Health Promotion in a Globalized World (WHO, 2005) is seen as the first attempt to revise the Ottawa Charter and identifies actions, commitments and pledges required to address the *determinants of health* in a globalized world through health promotion.

The Bangkok Charter 2005

Health promotion is the process of enabling people to increase control over their health and its determinants, and thereby improve their health. It is a core function of public health and contributes to the work of tackling communicable and non-communicable diseases and other threats to health (WHO, 2005).

The Bangkok Charter builds on the principles and action areas of the Ottawa Charter but is seen to be directed at the private sector and governments rather than a strategy for 'health promotion practitioners'. The Bangkok charter sets out five required actions that all sectors and settings must act upon: advocate; invest; build capacity; regulate and legislate and build alliances and partnerships. The Bangkok Charter recommends an integrated policy approach at national and international levels towards key commitments for the promotion of health:

- make the promotion of health central to global development agenda;
- make the promotion of health a core responsibility for all of government;
- make the promotion of health a key focus of communities and *civil society* and
- make the promotion of health a requirement fort good corporate practice.

Unlike the Ottawa Charter, the Bangkok Charter does not provide a framework that health promotion practitioners can use to directly help to enable their clients to take control over the influences on their health. The Bangkok Charter is intended for a different audience, governments and politicians at all levels, the private sector, international organizations as well as civil society and the public health community. The four commitments of the Bangkok Charter for Health Promotion in a Globalized World (WHO, 2005) are to make the promotion of health: central to the global development agenda; a core responsibility for all of government; a key focus on communities and civil society and a requirement for good corporate practice. These commitments require strong intergovernmental and corporate agreements and action. The experience of the Ottawa Charter has shown that social and political change (empowerment) has a better chance of success when it is backed by a 'movement' of professionals and civil society. It remains unclear who will be the 'champions' of the Bangkok Charter and who will back its development in the future.

A major obstacle in fulfilling the potential of health promotion has been its inability to close the implementation gap especially with regard to core concepts such as community empowerment. This was the key theme of the 7th Global Conference on Health Promotion (Promoting health and development: Closing the implementation gap) (WHO, 2009) held between 26th and 30th October 2009 in Nairobi, Kenya. The conference was a mammoth effort attended by over 600 invited experts from 100 countries. A key outcome of the conference was the Nairobi call to action that identifies key strategies and commitments urgently required for closing the implementation gap in health and development through health promotion. The main strategies and actions are presented under five sub-themes: building capacity or health promotion; strengthening health systems; partnerships and inter-sectoral action; community empowerment and health literacy and health behaviours. The call to action set out over 70 actions to close the implementation gap in health promotion. Some actions are broad such as 'by ensuring basic education for all citizens' others are specific such as 'by investing in research and *evaluation*, and its dissemination to increase the adoption of better practices in health promotion'. Some actions seem unrealistic such as 'by establishing good governance with respect to integrity, transparency and accessibility'. The broad range of actions covers all eventualities but could be confusing. The call to action required more direction, focus and a real practical purpose to directly address awkward political issues concerning the underlying health determinants rooted in poverty, *powerlessness* and inequality. The experience of the Ottawa Charter demonstrated that a strategic document has a better chance of success when it is backed by a 'movement' of professionals and civil society. For this to happen with the Nairobi call, a plan of action was required with clearly defined roles, responsibilities and timelines, but this has not happened. The WHO has also not issued an official statement, declaration or charter following the Nairobi 7th Global Conference on Health Promotion (Laverack, 2010).

KEY TEXTS

- World Health Organization (2009a) *Milestones in Health Promotion: Statements from Global Conferences* (Geneva: World Health Organization)
- World Health Organization (1986) *The Ottawa Charter for Health Promotion* (Geneva: World Health Organization)
- World Health Organization (2005) *The Bangkok Charter for Health Promotion in a Globalized World. 6th Global Conference on Health Promotion* (Geneva: World Health Organization)

definition

SEE ALSO **community capacity building; competencies; declarations and statements; health education; theories and models**

Health promotion is a contested concept and there is no singularly accepted definition. However, it can be regarded 'to represent a comprehensive social and political process, embracing actions directed at strengthening the skills and capabilities of individuals, and actions directed at changing social, environmental and economic conditions so as to alleviate their impact on health' (WHO, 1998, p. 1).

Broadly defined, health promotion aims to enable people to take more control over the determinants of their lives and health. Health promotion is both a set of principles involving equity, compassion and *empowerment* and a practice encompassing a range of communication, capacity building, training and politically orientated activities. Health promoters increase the assets and attributes of their clients (individuals, groups, organizations and communities) to gain more control over decisions and resources regarding the determinants of their health. Individual and collective empowerment are both central to this process and to health promotion theory and practice. The concept of empowerment has even been formalized in two of its key charters: the Ottawa Charter for Health Promotion (WHO, 1986) and the Bangkok Charter for Health Promotion in a Globalized World (WHO, 2005). In twenty years, between the publication of the Ottawa Charter in 1986 and later the Bangkok Charter in 2005, the core theme in health promotion has remained unchanged. This is the process of empowerment in which the practitioner acts as a facilitator to assist their clients to gain more *power*.

Health promotion practice is set within the design of an intervention, a project or a programme, most often controlled by government departments, agencies or government-funded non-governmental organizations. Health promotion practice is usually managed and monitored by a practitioner and addresses prioritized concerns that are then reflected as a statement of objectives, identifying in advance suitable indicators of progress and the assessment of risks. Within a practice context, there is always some power relationship between different people, primarily between practitioners and their clients. Practitioners are employed to deliver information, resources and services and are often seen as an outside agent to the people who benefit from the programme. Practitioners call themselves 'health promoters' or 'public health workers', while many more who look to the idea of health promotion occupy roles such as nurses, environmental health officers, housing officers and doctors. Their 'clients' cover the range of people with whom they work including women, adolescents, the homeless, men and other professional groups (Laverack, 2005).

The term 'supportive environments' is used in some definitions *of* health promotion as the protection of people from threats to health, and to enable people to expand their capabilities and develop self-reliance in health. They encompass where people live, their local *community*, their home, where they work and play, including people's access to resources for health and opportunities for *empowerment*. Action to create supportive environments for health has many dimensions, and may include direct political action to develop and implement policies and regulations that help create supportive environments, economic action, particularly in relation to fostering sustainable economic development and social action (WHO, 1998, p. 20).

Infrastructure for health promotion refers to those human and material resources, organizational and administrative structures, policies, regulations and incentives, which facilitate an organized response to health issues and challenges. Such infrastructures may be found through a diverse range of organizational structures, including *primary health care*, government, private sector and non-governmental organizations, self-help organizations, as well as dedicated health promotion agencies and *foundations*. Although many countries have a dedicated health promotion workforce, the greater human resource is to be found among the wider health workforce and in sectors other than health, for example, in education and social welfare, and from the actions of lay persons within *civil society*. Infrastructure for health promotion can be found not only in tangible resources and structures, but also through the extent of public and political awareness of health issues, and participation in action to address those issues (WHO, 1998, p. 14).

There is sometimes confusion about the differences between the definition of health promotion and *health education*. The most practical way forward is to view health promotion as encompassing health education as a range of educational and awareness raising activities.

While health promotion remains a contested concept with many interpretations and no singularly accepted definition, in practice it is often the World Health definitions stated in the Ottawa and Bangkok charters that are most likely to be cited. These can be summarized as 'health promotion is the process of enabling people to increase control over, and to improve, their health and its determinants.'

KEY TEXTS

- Ewles, L. and Simnett, I. (2009) *Promoting Health: A Practical Guide.* 5th edn (London: Bailliere Tindall)
- Keleher, H., Mac Dougall, C. and Murphy, B. (2007) *Understanding Health Promotion* (Melbourne: Oxford University Press)
- Tones, K. and Green, J. (2004) *Health Promotion: Planning and Strategies* (London: Sage Publications)

determinants of health

SEE ALSO civil society; lifestyle approach; social justice

The determinants of health encompass the economic and social conditions that influence the health of individuals, communities and populations. The social determinants of health are the conditions in which people are born, grow, live, work and age, circumstances that are shaped by the distribution of money, *power* and resources and which are themselves influenced by policy choices (WHO, 2008).

The determinants of health may seem distant to an individual or a *community*, but they nonetheless exert enormous influence over their everyday lives. The determinants of health gained prominence in the late 1980s and are the range of personal, economic and environmental factors, which 'determine' the health status of individuals and populations. The social determinants of health provide a direct political link to health promotion, *powerlessness* and inequality. Addressing the determinants of health requires, in part, an approach that moves towards an approach that posits health as being determined by how societies themselves are structured (Mouy and Barr, 2006).

The way in which society is structured, institutionalized and the inequities that this can create are not seen as a key part of the causes of poor health. Instead, health issues such as drug abuse, homelessness and social exclusion continue to be primarily viewed as problems of individual lifestyles. The health of the poor, the social gradient in health within countries and the marked health inequities between countries are caused by the unequal distribution of power, income, goods and services. The inequalities that this creates in everyday living include unequal access to health care and education, conditions of work and the limited opportunities of leading a healthy life. This unequal distribution is the result of a combination of poor social policies and programmes, unfair economic arrangements and unjust governance. People who have, for example, high-risk lifestyles or who have poor living conditions are typically more influenced by economic and political policies, suffer greater health inequalities and consequently have more disease, premature death and less well-being (Wilkinson, 2003). Health status improves at each step up the income and social hierarchy. The *social gradient* in health means that health inequities affect everyone especially the poorest of the poor, around the world, who have the worst health. Within countries, the lower an individual's socioeconomic position the worse their health (WHO, 2008). Prominent researchers such as Professor Sir Michael Marmot have claimed that *social injustice* and health inequalities are killing people on a grand scale because of the social gradient and the imbalances in the distribution of power, money and resources that it represents (Marmot, Allen and Goldblatt, 2010).

The Commission on Social Determinants of Health (CSDH) was established in 2005 to provide advice on how to reduce health inequalities and its final report contained three overarching recommendations (WHO, 2008):

1. Tackle the inequitable distribution of power, money and resources.

The key to addressing the determinants of and inequalities in health is through the redistribution of power and by transforming unequal power relationships, which are indicative of our society and working practices. Inequity in the conditions of daily living is shaped by deeper social structures and processes and is produced by social norms, policies and practices that tolerate or actually promote unfair distribution of and access to power, wealth and other necessary social resources.

2. Measure and understand the problem and assess the impact of action.

Action on the social determinants of health will be more effective if basic data systems, including vital registration and routine monitoring of health inequity and the social determinants of health, are put in place so that more effective policies, systems and programmes can be developed.

3. Improve daily living conditions.

Improving daily living conditions through the social determinants of health is an integral part of health programmes and an essential requirement for most people suffering poverty and powerlessness. The inequities in how society is organized mean that the freedom to enjoy good health is unequally distributed between and within societies. This inequity is seen in the conditions of early childhood and schooling, the nature of employment and working conditions, the physical form of the built environment and the quality of the natural environment in which people reside. Depending on the nature of these environments, different groups will have different experiences of material conditions, social support and opportunity, which make them more or less likely to suffer poorer health.

The daily conditions in which people live have a strong influence on health equity. Access to quality housing and clean water and sanitation are human rights. Broad policy interventions related to healthy urbanization include stimulation of job creation, land tenure and land use policy, transportation, sustainable urban development, social protection, settlement policies, slum upgrading and better security. Employment and working conditions have powerful effects on health equity. When these are good, they can provide financial security, social status, personal development, social relations and self-esteem and protection from physical and psychosocial illness. A good diet and an adequate supply of food, for example, are basic but important to *health and wellbeing*. A poor diet can cause malnutrition and a variety of deficiencies that can contribute to, for example, cancer and diabetes and can also lead to obesity (WHO, 2008).

The Commission on Social Determinants of Health was made up of nineteen experienced members, mostly academics, with the power to make independent recommendations. However, the Commission's report did not make a strong political statement by naming the perpetrators of social injustice or by stating the actions necessary to deal with them. Instead it presented the evidence of the 'causes of the causes' and recommended more and better research (Laverack, 2012). However, health promotion practice does not need more of the same research to describe the problem; it needs effective reforms and interventions to act on and solve health inequalities (Potvin, 2009).

KEY TEXTS
- Marmot, M. and Wilkinson, R.G. (2005) *Social Determinants of Health* (Oxford: Oxford University Press)
- Nathanson, C. and Hopper, K. (2010) 'The Marmot Review-Social Revolution by Stealth', *Social Science and Medicine*, 71: pp. 1237–1239
- World Health Organization (2008) *Closing the Gap in a Generation*. Commission on Social Determinants of Health. Final Report (Geneva: World Health Organization) www.who.int/social_determinants [accessed 6/5/2012]

disease prevention

SEE ALSO **approaches; behaviour change communication; hygiene promotion; lifestyle approach; risk factors; screening**

Disease prevention covers measures not only to prevent the occurrence of disease but also to arrest its progress and reduce its consequences once established. Disease prevention deals with individuals and populations identified as exhibiting identifiable *risk factors*, often associated with different risk behaviours (WHO, 1998, p. 4).

Health promotion is often categorized as being concerned with the primary, secondary and tertiary stages of disease prevention. Primary prevention is directed towards preventing the initial onset of ill health by, for example, the detection of risk factors, counselling and the appropriate health advice. Secondary prevention seeks to change unhealthy behaviour or to shorten the period of ill health and its progression, for example, educational and motivational strategies to increase physical activity or stress reduction. Tertiary prevention seeks to limit the effects of a chronic condition and enhance a person's quality of life, for example, effective rehabilitation therapy (Naidoo and Wills, 2009).

Chronic disease (also called non-communicable disease) prevention covers measures to prevent the occurrence of chronic disease, to arrest its progress and to reduce its consequences once established. Chronic disease is the world's leading cause of mortality. It persists over a long time and is most prevalent, but not exclusive to, the aged population (over 65 years of age). The risk of chronic disease is increased by certain 'risk factors' often caused by poor lifestyle choices such as tobacco use, lack of physical activity, poor eating habits, obesity and substance abuse. In turn, these factors can lead to obesity, hypertension, high cholesterol and increased vulnerability to stress. The leading chronic diseases in developed countries include arthritis, autoimmune diseases, heart attacks, strokes, cancers, diabetes and oral health problems (WHO, 2002; WHO, 2013). Many of these chronic diseases can be detected at an early stage of development.

Chronic disease prevention interventions focus on changing people's behaviour so that they will adopt a healthier lifestyle, for example, behaviour change strategies that promote good nutrition, smoking cessation and the moderate intake of alcohol. Classic examples of chronic disease prevention interventions include the North Karelia Project on cardiovascular disease (Puska *et al.*, 1995), the Multiple Risk Factors Intervention Trial (MRFIT) and the Community Intervention Trials for Smoking Cessation (COMMIT) (Syme, 1997). Despite their popularity, chronic disease prevention interventions have received criticism for their small degree of success relative to the resources expended. The most notable success has been with the educated and economically advantaged in society, for example, between 1998 and 2004, there was a 9% decrease in smoking in the lowest quintile in Australia compared to a 35% decrease in the highest quintile (Baum, 2007). As a consequence, some chronic disease prevention interventions may have had little effect in closing the gap between the 'healthy wealthy' at the top of the social gradient and low socio-economic groups further down the gradient. They may even, at least temporarily, have led to an increase in health inequalities (Baum, 2007). Australia's 'Swap it, don't swap' campaign, for example, used a character called 'Eric', a blue balloon-type figure, who urges others to swap unhealthy aspects of their lifestyle, such as physical inactivity, for healthier lifestyle habits. However, the changes necessary for 'Eric' to lead a healthier life actually required a change in the structures in which he lives, such as a safe neighbourhood (Baum, 2011). A political commitment to address the broader *determinants of health* only then to shift to a much narrower lifestyle intervention is a political trend that has been termed the 'lifestyle drift'.

The term 'obesogenic environment' refers to an environment that promotes gaining weight and one that is not conducive to weight loss within various *settings* such as the workplace or the community and therefore contributes to obesity. For example, if a community has cracked sidewalks, unkempt parks, a high crime rate and/or limited recreational opportunities, residents are less likely to engage in physical activity. Providing support at the community and policy level would include measures to improve the 'built environment', easier access to healthy foods and facilities and community to promote physically active (Swinburn, Eggar and Raza, 1999).

Communicable disease (also called infectious and transmissible disease) prevention covers measures to prevent the occurrence of communicable disease, to arrest its progress and to reduce its consequences once established. Communicable diseases comprise clinically evident illnesses resulting from the infection, presence and growth of pathogenic and biological agents in an individual. Infectious pathogens include some viruses, bacteria, fungi, protozoa and parasites. An infectious disease is transmitted from some source, such as from one person to another or from a vector such as an animal to a person. Defining the means of transmission plays an important part in understanding the biology of an infectious agent and in addressing the disease it causes.

Communicable disease prevention interventions focus on controlling or eliminating the cause of transmission, the vector or the high-risk behaviour. In some cases, this can be done using a physical method, for example, a mosquito bed-net or chemical spray for malaria control or a condom for preventing the spread of a sexually transmitted disease. For other infectious diseases, a vaccine can be used to reduce the effect such as for measles. Examples of communicable disease prevention interventions include malaria and dengue control, *hygiene promotion* to prevent the spread of intestinal parasites and diarrhoeal diseases and the promotion of behaviour change to combat sexually transmitted diseases.

The systematic, ongoing collection, collation and analysis of health-related information that is communicated in a timely manner to all who need to know which health problems require action is used for both chronic and communicable disease prevention. However, surveillance and *screening* is particularly important with communicable disease prevention because of the infectious nature of certain organisms and the rapid spread of disease that can result in the population. Information that is used for surveillance comes from many sources, including reported cases of communicable diseases, hospital admissions, laboratory reports, population surveys, reports of absence from school or work and reported causes of death (PHAC, 2013).

KEY TEXTS
- Woolf, S., Jonas, S. and Kaplan-Liss, E. (2007) *Health Promotion and Disease Prevention in Clinical Practice* (Philadelphia: Lippincott Williams and Wilkins)
- World Health Organization (2002) *The World Health Report 2002 – Reducing Risks, Promoting Healthy Life* (Geneva: World Health Organization)
- World Health Organization (2013) *Chronic Diseases and Health Promotion.* http://www.who.int/chp/en/

e

empowerment

SEE ALSO approaches; community capacity building; definition; gender and health; health activism; power; theory and models

Empowerment in the broadest sense is '...the process by which disadvantaged people work together to increase control over events that determine their lives' (Werner, 1988, p. 1).

Most definitions of empowerment give the term a similarly positive value, and have been largely developed in western and uniquely American value systems, which place strong emphasis individual and *community* responsibility (Minkler, 1989). They embody the notion that empowerment must come from within an individual, group or community and cannot be given to them. It is through the process of community empowerment that people are best able to achieve the broader social and political change that is necessary to improve their lives and health. To provide clarity to this concept, it is useful to consider the different levels of community empowerment. Christopher Rissel (1994, p. 1) includes a heightened or an increased level of psychological empowerment as a part of community empowerment and argues that it includes '...a political action component in which members have actively participated, and the achievement of some redistribution of resources or decision making favourable to the community or group in question.' Barbara Israel and her colleagues (1994) similarly identify psychological and political action as two levels of community empowerment, but include a third, and intermediary level between them, that of organizational empowerment. Their analysis of this level draws heavily from democratic management theory. An empowered organization is one that is democratically managed, and its members share information and control over decisions and are involved in the design, implementation and control of efforts towards goals defined by group consensus. It is an essential link

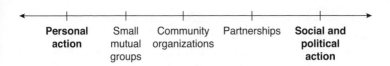

FIGURE I   *The Community Empowerment Continuum*

between empowered individuals and effective political action and is similar to the structure of many *pressure groups* and social movements.

Community empowerment includes personal empowerment, family empowerment, organizational empowerment and broader social and political changes. It is a dynamic process involving continual shifts in personal empowerment and changes in *power* relations between different social groups and decision makers in the broader society (Laverack, 2004). Community empowerment outcomes include the redistribution of resources, a decrease in *powerlessness* or success in achieving social and political change. However, it is as a process that it is most consistently viewed in the literature, for example, '... a social-action process that promotes participation of people, organizations and communities towards the goals of increased individual and community control, political efficacy, improved quality of life and social justice' (Wallerstein, 1992, p. 1). As a process, community empowerment is best considered as a continuum representing progressively more organized and broadly based forms of collective action.

Each point on the continuum can be viewed as a progression towards the goals of social and political action. The groups and organizations that develop in the process have their own dynamics, they may flourish for a time then fade away, for reasons as much to do with changes in the community as with a lack of broader political or financial support. The weakness of the continuum approach is that it offers a simple, linear interpretation of what can be a more fluid and complex process. Nonetheless, the continuum provides a valuable tool to help practitioners to understand how they can become involved in empowering *approaches*. The role of the practitioner is as a 'facilitator' to support and enable individuals, groups and communities to progress along the continuum. The desired outcomes are actions that bring about social and political change. Social change refers to societal norms, beliefs and behaviours that have an influence on the community. In turn, the political change refers to policy, legislation and governance that have a direct influence on people's health (Labonte and Laverack, 2008).

Gaining power to influence economic, political, social and ideological change will inevitably involve the community in a struggle with those already holding power. The role of the health promoting agency, at the request of the community, is to build capacity, provide resources and to help to empower individuals and organizations. Working in empowering ways is also a *political activity* because the structures of power-over, of bureaucracy and authority that create powerlessness remain dominant. The role of health promotion is to strive to help others to challenge these circumstances.

KEY TEXTS
- Kendall, S. (ed) (1998) *Health and Empowerment: Research and Practice* (London: Arnold Publications)
- Laverack, G. (2004) *Health Promotion Practice: Power and Empowerment* (London: Sage Publications)
- Laverack, G. (2007) *Health Promotion Practice: Building Empowered Communities* (Maidenhead: Open University Press)

ethics

SEE ALSO **competencies; definition; evaluation; powerlessness**

Ethics is a branch of philosophy dealing with distinctions between right and wrong, and with the moral consequences of human actions. Much of modern ethical thinking is based on the concepts of human rights, individual freedom and autonomy, and on doing good and not harming (PHAC, 2013).

There is a good deal of discussion regarding the application of ethics to health promotion including a lively critical disassembling of definitions and models that suffused the 1980s and 1990s. It is possible to follow four simple points for an ethical approach to health promotion that combine a blend of liberalism (provision of core resources but not a guarantee of full equality), utilitarianism (improve these core conditions for all rather than for particular 'groups') and egalitarianism (make this improvement a social priority for all) (Seedhouse, 1997). The four points for an ethical approach to health promotion are as follows:

- a core respect for the autonomy of individuals;
- a focus on central conditions in people's lives that support such autonomy;
- prevention of disease, illness, injury and disability as legitimate health 'targets' and
- the prevention of obstacles in achieving the aforementioned three points.

Central to an ethical approach to health promotion is *empowerment*. Per-Anders Tengland (2007) believes that the logic for using an empowering approach in health promotion is justified because it is well founded and ethically and morally sound to do so. Tengland concludes from a conceptual analysis that as a means or as a process empowerment has applicability for creating freedom and opportunity to improve health. However, he questions whether most practitioners have the knowledge and skills that are required to undertake an ethical approach to their work in health promotion. Practitioners often work with people from different cultural backgrounds and need to have a shared understanding if they are to use empowering *approaches* in their everyday work. This would include a better understanding of themselves, their beliefs and values and to put this into a framework of the relevant social and cultural perceptions.

A key ethical tension in health promotion practice is whether people actually want to gain more control over their lives, health and its determinants. It is the practitioner, or their agency, that usually initiates the health promotion project and provides the initial enthusiasm for its direction. This is contradictory to an empowering approach in which the issue to be addressed and the means of reaching a solution should be the responsibility of the beneficiaries of the programme, based on their informed or intuitive needs. Some people may simply not want to be involved. People, especially if they have lived in oppressive or powerless circumstances, may feel that they do not have the right or do not possess the motivation to empower themselves.

Do people have a right not to become empowered? It must be remembered that *power* cannot be given but people must gain or seize it for themselves. The right to be empowered rests with the individual or group and the role of the practitioner is to facilitate and enable others to take greater responsibility and control over their lives. Some people may not want the responsibility of making decisions or fear the regret of making a misjudgement and therefore 'delegate' this authority to another person in whom they have trust. Other individuals, for example, the very young, the very old or people with an addiction, may not have the ability to sufficiently organize and mobilize themselves collectively. For those who cannot or who refuse to take responsibility, health practice may have to intervene and resort to a more paternalistic approach, for example, through policy and legislation to prevent the spread of an infectious disease, to protect population health or place an individual into care (even against their wishes) to ensure the wellbeing of themselves. Other examples are the enforcement of speed limits to protect drivers and pedestrians and legislation to restrict the sale of alcohol and tobacco to children (Baum, 2008).

Key ethical issues raised in health promotion practice are behaviour modification and include strong paternalism, coercion and manipulation and, in particular, not respecting personal autonomy. Autonomy refers to the capacity to be self-governing, to making the decisions that will influence one's life and health. It is linked to what it is to be a person, to be able to choose freely and to be able to formulate how one wants to live one's life. It is also related to having the freedom and opportunities in our lives to be able to make the right choices for ourselves (Kant, 2004). Another ethical issue refers to 'blaming'. The assumption that changing knowledge would also lead to a change in a person's attitude and practice, for example, with regard to eating healthily. This is paternalistic and places an emphasis on individual responsibility when it is wrong to think that people are free to choose healthier options because other factors that determine their behaviour may be out of their control, for example, being unemployed or homeless (Holland, 2007). However, those defined as 'victims' may sometimes identify themselves with this term and feel that they do not have the right or do not possess the motivation to change their circumstances. This has been applied to people living in risk conditions when individuals internalize *powerlessness* creating a potent psychological barrier to action. They accept aspects of their world that are self-destructive to their own wellbeing, thinking that these are unalterable features of what they take to be 'reality', a condition called surplus powerlessness (Lerner, 1986).

In conclusion, how best to apply ethical principles to health promotion is unresolved and remains a matter of some academic debate (Holland, 2007).

KEY TEXTS

- Anand, S., Fabienne, P. and Sen, A. (2006) *Public Health, Ethics and Equity* (Oxford: Oxford University Press)
- Cribb, A. and Duncan, P. (2002) *Health Promotion and Professional Ethics* (Oxford: Blackwell Publishing)
- Holland, S. (2007) *Public Health Ethics* (Cambridge, UK: Polity Press)

evaluation

SEE ALSO **approaches; bottom-up and top-down; ethics; evidence-based practice; health profiles; theory and models**

Health promotion evaluation is an assessment of the extent to which health promotion actions achieve a valued outcome (WHO, 1998, p. 12).

While there is no real agreement about the overall purpose of evaluation in a health promotion programme context, it should address the overall health goals that reflect the values of the *community*, in general, and the health sector, in particular, regarding a healthy society. The evaluation should also address the concerns of the programme stakeholders who require information about its impact, operation, progress and achievements. Evaluation is an integral part of management (Usher, 1995), with the purpose of providing inputs to ongoing activities and information for the future design and the effectiveness (have I met my targets) and efficiency (the outcomes in relation to the inputs). Evaluation also has a role in the accountability of programmes usually to an outside agency that contributes to the funding (Rebien, 1996). In top-down programming, evaluation can be used as an instrument of control through performance measurement in terms of achieving targets by providing feedback about the operational elements of the programme implementation. The evaluation typically uses predetermined indicators, towards which the primary stakeholders do not contribute, and is often implemented by a health promotion 'expert'. The role of the health promoter as an outside agent has been traditionally viewed as one of 'expert', one who judges merit or worth (Patton, 1997). Bottom-up programming places the focus on the process towards participatory self-evaluation and away from conventional 'expert'-driven *approaches*. This means a fundamental shift in the *power* relationship between the outside agents and the beneficiaries of the programme, one where control over decisions about design and evaluation is more equitably distributed. The evaluation helps to empower the beneficiaries by actively involving them in the process and by subsequently providing the means to make decisions to improve their lives and health (Laverack, 2007).

Two ideal paradigms that are relevant to the evaluation of health promotion are positivist and constructivist. A paradigm can be defined as a world view that is composed of multiple belief categories, principal among them being their ontological, epistemological and methodological assumptions. Ontological assumptions are about the way in which the world is, the nature of reality. Epistemological assumptions are about what we can know about that reality. Methodological assumptions are about how we come to know that reality and the strategies we employ in order to discover the way in which the world functions (Guba, 1990). The conventional health promotion paradigm is typified as the positivist approach. Its ontology consists of a belief in a single reality, independent of any observer and a belief that universal truths independent of time and place exist and can be discovered. Its epistemology consists of a belief that the evaluator can and should investigate a phenomenon in a way that is uncluttered by values and biases. The methodology of the conventional paradigm favours experimental designs to test hypotheses and is concerned with prediction through proof or certainty and with singular measures of reality and truth (Labonte and Robertson, 1996). The constructivist approach provides a wider framework in which 'truth' and 'fact' are recognized for having subjective dimensions. What emerges from this process is an agenda for negotiation based on the issues raised during dialogue between the evaluator and those with who they are involved in the evaluation. Its ontology is relativist, meaning that realities are socially constructed. Realities are local and specific, dependent on their form and content and on the persons who hold them. Its epistemology recognizes the evaluator as part of the reality that is being evaluated and the findings are a creation of the inquiry process between the inquirer and inquired. Individual constructions are elicited, refined, compared and contrasted, with the aim of generating one or more constructions on which there is substantial consensus. In the constructivist paradigm, truth is not absolute, but rather is understood as the best informed and most sophisticated truth we might construct at any given moment. This paradigm seeks to know by understanding how and what people experience within their context and its application in health promotion programmes (Labonte and Robertson, 1996).

The accountability and effectiveness of health promotion is an on-going discussion, often in association with the use of an evidence-based approach. Health promoters are increasingly being asked to provide greater evidence of their work, even though the theories, models and approaches that they use are often contested and considered to be untested (Raphael, 2000). *Evidence-based* practice involves the judgements of both practitioners and their clients and a systematic appraisal of research, *theory and models* (NSW Government, 2013).

Formative evaluation is used to assess how the programme works: Is it being delivered effectively for the purpose of improving the way it is offered? Summative evaluation is used to assess the outcome of the programme to determine whether or not the goals have been achieved, especially in relation to policy and budget decision making (Jirojwong and Liamputtong, 2009). However, it can be difficult to trace the pathways that link particular health promotion outcomes to specific health outcomes such as a reduction in morbidity and mortality, BMI or a reduction in hypertension. In a bio-medically dominated profession, this can result in a diminished value being attributed to the role of health promotion programmes. Confounding factors and technical difficulties of isolating cause and effect in complex lifestyle situations require health promoters to set realistic and relevant goals, outcomes and targets for their work (WHO, 1998).

Bamberger, Rugh and Mabry (2006) provide a simple approach that capture the essence of the process of evaluation and places an emphasis on methodological rigour in health promotion programmes. The first step is planning and scoping the evaluation, followed by strategies to address the budget constraints of the programme. The evaluation must also take into account any time constraints of a new or on-going programme and problems for collecting data. The issue of political influences in the design, implementation and dissemination of the findings is sometimes not considered by health promoters but is an important step in the evaluation process. The dissemination, validation and use of the information gained from the evaluation is an especially neglected area by many health promotion programmes. Important findings can be lost in the grey literature and are not effectively used in improving future programme design, policy or budget allocation for improving health. Bamberger, Rugh and Mabry (2006) rightfully advocate for special attention and additional resources and time to be allocated to the utilization of the evaluation findings. It is crucial that health promoters are sensitive to the position of their work and the influence that this can have on their clients. Such awareness is termed a reflexive practice. A reflexive health promotion practice allows practitioners to be critical about the way they use their knowledge and power to have professional influence over others, including other professionals and their clients (Laverack, 2009, p. 61).

The broader debate regarding health promotion evaluation encompasses the underlying philosophy, principles and values, professional *competencies*, the role of community-led participatory approaches, accountability to policy makers and cause and effect in complex situations. At a pragmatic level, the evaluation of health promotion focuses on the use of an evidence-based approach and on the need to use realistic outcomes in a programme context. Health promotion outcomes are changes to personal characteristics and skills, and/ or social norms and actions and/or organizational practices and public policies, which are attributable to a health promotion activity. Health promotion outcomes represent the most immediate results of health promotion activities including *health literacy, healthy public policy* and community action for health.

A health outcome is a change in the health status of an individual, group or population, which is attributable to a planned intervention, regardless of whether or not such an intervention was intended to change health status. Health outcomes are usually assessed using health indicators, a characteristic that can be used to describe one or more measurable aspects of the health of an individual or population (quality, quantity) over time, such as the programme period. Health indicators may include the measurement of illness or disease, or positive aspects of health (such as quality of life, *life skills* or health expectancy) and of behaviours and actions that are related to healthy lifestyles such as exercise and smoking. They may also include indicators that measure the social and economic conditions and the physical environment as it relates to health, measures of health literacy and healthy public policy. This latter group of indicators may be used to measure intermediate health outcomes, health targets and health promotion outcomes (WHO, 1998).

Intermediate health outcomes are changes in the *determinants of health*, notably changes in lifestyles, and living conditions that are attributable to a planned intervention such as health promotion, *disease prevention* and *primary health care*. Health targets also state, for a given population, the amount of change that could be reasonably expected within a defined time period as an assessment of progress in relation to a defined health policy or programme. This is in relation to a defined benchmark against which progress can be measured. Setting targets requires the existence of a relevant health indicator and information on the distribution of that indicator within a population of interest. *Health profiles*, for example, provide a summary of health information for a particular population and sub-divided into regions, provinces, towns and local communities. Health profiles are used to help prioritize and plan services including health promotion (Network of Public Health Observatories, 2013). Health targets also require an estimate of current and likely future trends in relation to change in the distribution of the indicator, and an understanding of the potential to change the distribution of the indicator in the population (WHO, 1998).

The evaluation of health promotion is an evolving field with an urgent need to provide more evidence of what really works in practice. This is made more difficult because of the wide range of approaches, models and theories that are used in health promotion and the overlap and lack of clarity that occurs between them.

Advances in an evidence-based approach for the effectiveness of both top-down and bottom-up programmes would make a real contribution to health promotion practice and to the role of practitioners (Rootman *et al.*, 2001).

KEY TEXTS

- Green, J. and South, J. (2006) *Evaluation* (Maidenhead: Open University Press)
- Hubley, J., Copeman, J. and Woodall, J. (2013) *Practical Health Promotion*. 2nd edn (Cambridge, UK: Polity Press)
- Nutbeam, D. and Bauman, A (2006) *Evaluation in a Nutshell* (Sydney, Australia: McGraw-Hill Book Company)
- Rootman, I. *et al.* (2001) *Evaluation in Health Promotion: Principles and Perspectives*. Series Number 92 (Copenhagen: WHO European Office)
- Valente, T.W. (2002) *Evaluating Health Promotion Programs* (Oxford: Oxford University Press)

evidence-based practice

SEE ALSO **advocacy; competencies; evaluation; healthy public policy; needs assessment**

Evidence-based health promotion practice specifically refers to 'the development, implementation, and *evaluation* of effective programmes and policies through application of evidence, including systematic appraisal of research and appropriate use of programme planning models' (NSW Government, 2013).

Evidence-based practice, in whatever professional context, involves not only evidence but also the judgement (knowledge and experience) of the practitioner and also of their clients (Craig and Smyth, 2002). The movement to develop 'evidence-based practice' first began in the field of medicine but quickly spread to other parts of the health sector including health promotion. The movement addresses the integration of systematically derived knowledge with the practitioner's own experience and their interpretation of the needs of the people with whom they work.

Health promoters are increasingly being asked to justify what they do by providing evidence of effectiveness and it is now widely accepted that their activities should be supported by sound evidence. However, much of what counts as evidence in health promotion is a contested issue (Raphael, 2000), partly because it is not always possible to measure the important aspects of health promotion work. In the absence of empirical evidence, the profession has used other terms such as 'best practice' to suggest something that is more practicable. 'Best practice' refers to the body of literature covering the knowledge, tools and strategies, which have been evaluated and are accepted as being effective in health promotion. The impetus to broaden the health promotion agenda has been reinforced by concerns about the variable effectiveness of past health promotion initiatives and the increased understanding of growing inequalities in health. The development of evidence-based health promotion practice must therefore be examined in the light of the growing impetus for interventions that address environmental and contextual *determinants of health*, in addition to individuals' behavioural *risk factors* (Rychetnik and Wise, 2004).

The challenges of an evidence-based health promotion practice include having the availability of information from existing research and evaluation, statistical sources and expert knowledge. Evidence-based knowledge is not comprehensive and there are gaps in the research about the effectiveness of what health promoters do in their daily work. Evidence-based practice relies on the findings of research to be transferable into the work setting, but this is not necessarily the case, neither are practitioners skilled to appraise what works and what does not work for their professional context. For example, practitioners working with smokers in low-income communities need to understand the importance that smoking plays in some people's lives. Even when the person understands the health risks associated with smoking, this behaviour can be important to help them cope with living in poverty or being unemployed (Craig and Smyth, 2002). However, there are still those who would argue that either with or without an evidence base, health promotion is justified because it is ethical and principled and uses a value-based approach that is effective (Raphael, 2000).

There are several organizations that are involved in the assessment of the effectiveness of health promotion interventions including the Cochrane collaboration that facilitates accessibility to systematic reviews of the effects of health care and population health and the National Institute for Health and Clinical Excellence

(NICE) that supports evidence-based practice in clinical and population health.

KEY TEXTS

- Craig, J. and Smyth, R. (2002) *The Evidence-Based Practice Manual for Nurses* (Edinburgh: Churchill Livingstone)
- The Cochrane Collaboration, http://www.cochrane.org/ [accessed 15/3/2013]
- The National Institute for Health and Clinical Excellence, http://www.nice.org.uk. [accessed 15/3/2013]
- Perkins, E., Simnett, I. and Wright, L. (1999) *Evidence Based Health Promotion* (London: Wiley)

f

foundations

SEE ALSO alliances, partnerships and coalitions; competencies; networks

The development of Health Promotion Foundations has been an innovative way of mobilizing new resources for promoting health, to support research and to strengthen links with other sectors including education, sport, the arts and the environment. Health Promotion Foundations are essentially organizations that not only have unique features but that also share a number of common characteristics:

1. Health Promotion Foundations are established according to some form of legislation that defines their role in terms of its functions, objectives and powers and provides a recurrent budget.
2. Health Promotion Foundations are governed by an independent Board of Governance that comprise stakeholder representation and usually a mix of government and non-government organizations (NGOs), for example, representation from government or people with expertise in health and other sectors. Board members may also be nominated for their expertise in marketing, finance, *community* development or research.
3. Staff coordinating the activities of the Health Promotion Foundation are organized in teams or areas according to health promotion topics, for example, healthy body weight team, or roles, for example, grant and sponsorship.
4. Health Promotion Foundations promote health by working with and across many sectors and levels of society.
5. Health Promotion Foundations are not aligned with any one political group.

Health Promotion Foundations work strategically in the context of their country or state to set priorities that will be effective in achieving outcomes for health promotion. For example, 'Health Promotion Switzerland' works towards a long-term strategy (2007–2018), which has three core areas of focus: (1) strengthen health promotion and *disease prevention* through nationwide strategic activities and projects; (2) healthy body weight focus especially on the 1.8 million children and adolescents living in Switzerland and (3) workplace health promotion through the implementation of national wide projects.

Effective models for Health Promotion Foundations now exist in several countries including in Switzerland, Thailand, Tonga, Australia, Austria and Korea. A key mechanism for financing Health Promotion Foundations is through a dedicated tax on a harmful product such as tobacco. For example, the 'Thaihealth' Foundation is an independent state agency and is funded by a 2% surcharge tax of tobacco and alcohol excise taxes in the country. A hypothecation of tax enables the replacement of company sponsorship and support for a range of health promotion actions such as the prevention of cancer, injury and substance abuse (WHO, 2002). The WHO International Network of Health Promotion Foundations was established in 1999 to enhance their performance and to assist with the development of new Foundations.

KEY TEXTS

- Alchin, T.M. (1992) 'The Health Promotion Foundations: How Successful Are They?' *Working Papers in Economics* # wp. 92/03 (Sydney: University of Western Sydney)
- Health Promotion Foundations. http://www.hpfoundations.net/
- Network of Health Promotion Foundations. http://www.who.int/healthpromotion/areas/foundations/en/index.html
- Thai Health Promotion Foundation. http://en.thaihealth.or.th/

g

gender and health

SEE ALSO advocacy; boycotts; health social movements; power; powerlessness; pressure groups

The term 'gender' includes both masculinity and femininity. Being a man or a woman has a significant impact on health, as a result of biological and gender-related differences and factors such as poverty and *powerlessness*. Gender mainstreaming is an acknowledgement that gender equality is best achieved by integrating women's and men's health concerns aimed at improving health (WHO, 2013a).

Most health-related gender discussion over the past few decades has focussed on women's health needs because they were perceived as being the most disadvantaged. However, gender differences can also hurt men's health, for example, when greater risk-taking among young men leads to higher accident rates. Associating gender issues as the domain of women constrains the opportunities for developing men's health promotion as something that happens separately and independently of 'women's health' work. It also fails to recognize the key role that gender relations play in the generation of socially specific health practices for both men and women (Smith and Robertson, 2008).

Health promotion interventions for women's health have addressed a range of issues including reproductive and sexual health, maternal health, child care, the menopause, breast and ovarian cancer, osteoporosis and safety from domestic violence. Women have historically come together to share knowledge and experiences about their health and in particular feminist groups have also played an important role in this relationship. 'Code Pink', for example, is an international organization dedicated to uniting women against international and domestic violence. The group follows feminist ideals and advocates open and respectful communication and crea-tive unconventional tactics. Using the Internet, *media* coverage, pop culture and protests, Code Pink uses 'enjoyable' activism, including die-ins and teach-ins, offering highly visual events that attract media attention. Code Pink has also created a number of partnerships with other organizations, including those concerned with men's health, supporting peace and justice (Code Pink, 2012).

Advocacy has been a key strategy in the struggle for gender equality and for a commitment to non-discrimination and informed consent in health. This is because within society, both men and women often did not have the necessary right to make decisions about their own bodies. The women's health movement, for example, has always striven for their right to choose and be informed about better health options. The women's health movement was the force required to collectively organize and mobilize themselves towards addressing social injustice and inequalities. For example, the first birth-control pill was developed by men and tested on Puerto Rican women in the 1950s and did not become a prescription drug until the 1960s in the United States. Although it was initially met with enthusiasm, investigations by women's health groups exposed the risks of such a highly hormonal, and largely untested, fertility regimen and, more significantly, exposed the lack of information shared with women as patients, who took the pill every day. The pill remains a popular method and women are no longer expected to take instructions on the choice of contraception from medical professionals without question (Daly, 2007).

The narrow, discipline-specific understandings of men's health, spread across boundaries can be problematic for designing successful health promotion programmes. The focus has been on physical assessment and lifestyle advice, which fails to address wider issues impacting upon men's health practices in everyday life and also a tendency to utilize stereotypical aspects of masculinity as a way to draw men in to processes of engagement, for example, the 'pit-stop' program in Australia engages men by using analogies between car parts (Courtenay, 2011). An example of a men's health promotion project in a Canadian city focussed on male immigrants from Latin America. These men experienced the stresses of finding housing and work in a foreign culture, with a different language, often under the uncertainty of whether they would be able to stay permanently. They also smoked a lot and this caught the attention of a health department that initially used conventional strategies of education and awareness campaigns, designed in culturally and linguistically sensitive ways and marketed through channels, such as church and refugee assistance groups. However, *community* workers also knew that, until their lives and living conditions settled down, smoking would never be much of an issue for these men. Spanish-speaking health workers, still working to develop smoking awareness interventions, also asked the men about their greatest health worries. Consensus developed that their teenage children had nowhere to go and to combat drugs and petty crime they wanted to create a drop-in centre for Hispanic youth. In addition to conventional strategies, the project then started to address stress and the quality of men's participation in the centre as role models and leaders (Labonte, 1998).

Men's health promotion interventions have traditionally focussed on raising awareness of issues relating to young men and suicide, prostate disease, alcohol misuse, obesity, smoking, heart disease, stress and sexual health. However, more recently men's health policy has become more progressive by creating a policy environment that has required men's health advocates to work in partnership with women's health advocates. The rapid growth in the interest of men's health in the United Kingdom, for example, has stemmed in part from an increasingly strong and influential men's health movement, consisting of health professionals, academics and politicians (Courtenay, 2011).

Individual women and men have operated alone, largely or entirely independent of groups, for example, holding single-person vigils about health causes that society is unwilling to champion. Fathers 4 Justice (or F4J), for example, is a pressure group to champion the cause of equal parenting, family law reform and equal contact for male divorced parents with children. F4J members undertook a series of high-visibility stunts with the protesters often dressed as comic book superheroes and frequently climbing public buildings, bridges and monuments (Fathers4Justice, 2012). However, gender activists have been most successful when engaging collectively to change the structural and systemic causes of health inequalities. They have achieved these goals through their involvement in *pressure groups*, social networks and *health social movements*, by mobilizing resources and by improving their *competencies*. By operating collectively, they have benefited from sharing roles, responsibilities and expertise and by having a sense of solidarity for both men and women who might otherwise have felt isolated within society (Laverack, 2013).

KEY TEXTS

- Courtenay, W. (2011) *Dying to Be Men: Psychosocial, Environmental and Bio-Behavioural Directions in Promoting the Health of Men and Boys* (London: Routledge)
- Dubriwny, T. (2012) *The Vulnerable Empowered Woman: Feminism, Post Feminism and Women's Health (Critical Issues in Health and Medicine)* (Biggleswade, UK: Rutgers University Press)
- Sabo, D. and Gordon, D. (1995) *Men's Health and Illness: Gender, Power and the Body* (London: Sage Publications)
- Sargent, C.F. and Brettell, C. (1996) *Gender and Health: An International Perspective* (New Jersey: Prentice Hall)

global health

SEE ALSO **declarations and statements; disease prevention; public health**

Global health describes the entire population of the world including all nations with a cultural and territorial identity, states, as the political organizations of these nations, multi-national organizations and academic institutions involved with the production of knowledge related to global health issues (Parker and Sommer, 2011).

Populations face transnational impacts of globalization upon health determinants and problems that are beyond the control of individual nations (Lee, 2003). Issues on the global health agenda include the inequities caused by patterns of international trade and investment, the effects of global climate change, the vulnerability of refugee populations, the marketing of harmful products by transnational corporations and the transmission of diseases between countries. However, the concept that can best fit the challenges faced by global health is the global transfer of health risks as a result of an expansion of the movement of people, environmental threats, lifestyle changes, variance of health and safety standards and trade in harmful products (Parker and Sommer, 2011).

The distinction between global health issues and those that could be regarded as international health issues is that the former defy control by the institutions of individual countries. These global threats to health require partnerships for priority setting and health promotion at both the national and international level. Until recently, most health promoters, development agencies and non-governmental organizations mobilized themselves around 'international health' issues: the greater burden of disease faced by poor groups in poor countries. Health promoters working to reduce HIV prevalence in Africa, to improve maternal/child health programmes in Latin America or to create gender *empowerment* projects in South Asia were engaged in international health work. Their programmes were simply international extensions into other countries of the work they might have done within their own borders. The only 'global' component is that funding for this work was often provided through agencies based in industrialized countries, whether official or funnelled through NGOs, to aid in the health development of countries lagging behind (Labonte and Laverack, 2008).

Global health implies that no longer can health issues and their social determinants in one country be divorced from issues in another. Many health promotion issues are now situated within the context of globalization. These are the worldwide connections and *networks* of people and organizations that span national, geographic and cultural borders and boundaries (Naidoo and Wills, 2009). Globalization, at its simplest, describes a constellation of processes by which nations, businesses and people are becoming more connected and interdependent through increased economic integration and communication exchange, cultural diffusion and travel (Labonte and Laverack, 2008). Health promotion entered the globalization ideology debate somewhat late and is still in its infancy in coming to terms with its implications. The Bangkok Charter for Health Promotion in a Globalized World, for example, posits that health promotion must become 'central to the global development agenda'. While a reasonable claim, it does not, unfortunately, provide a clear role for practitioners or provide a plan of action indicating who, how and when this commitment will be achieved, apart from developing the role of partnerships. Health promotion must become an integral part of domestic and foreign policy and international relations, including in situations of war and conflict. This requires actions to promote dialogue and cooperation among nation states, *civil society* and the private sector (WHO, 2005).

KEY TEXTS

- Labonte, R. and Laverack, G. (2008) *Health Promotion in Action: From Local to Global Empowerment* (Basingstoke: Palgrave MacMillan)
- Lee, K. (2003) *Globalization and Health: An Introduction* (Basingstoke: Palgrave Macmillan)
- Parker, R. and Sommer, M. (2011) *Handbook in Global Public Health* (Abingdon: Routledge)

h

harm reduction

SEE ALSO **lifespan approach; lifestyle approach; mental health promotion; peer education; risk factors**

Harm reduction is a pragmatic approach to reduce the harmful consequences of high-risk behaviours by incorporating strategies that cover safer use, managed use and abstinence (Ritter and Cameron, 2006).

High risk behaviours that have been included in harm reduction interventions are needle exchange, opioid substitution therapy, substance use prevention for adolescents, smoking cessation, homelessness and sex work. The principles of harm reduction are often firmly rooted in humanistic ideals, in immediate and attainable goals and the recognition that risky behaviours have always been and always will be a part of society (Ritter and Cameron, 2006). The primary goal of most harm-reduction *approaches* is to work with individuals on their terms in their context and not to condemn their harmful behaviours. The goal is to work with the individual or *community* to minimize the harmful effects of a given behaviour. Unlike the moral approach of addiction, which tends to enhance the user's shame, guilt and feelings of stigma, the harm-reduction approach is based on acceptance and the willingness of the provider to collaborate with clients in the course of reducing harmful consequences (Marlatt and Witkiewitz, 2010).

Harm minimization is often used interchangeably with harm reduction. However, any intervention or policy that is intended to reduce harm and problem behaviour can be considered harm reducing. The term harm minimization is intended to reflect an overall goal of policies to minimize harm (Weatherburn, 2009).

An example of one harm reduction intervention used brief motivational interviews to reduce alcohol-related consequences among adolescents (aged 18–19 years) treated in an emergency room following an alcohol-related event. An assessment of their condition and future risk of harm and the motivational interviews were conducted in the emergency room during or after the patient's treatment. Follow-up assessments showed that patients who received the motivational interviews had a significantly lower incidence of drinking and driving, traffic violations, alcohol-related injuries and alcohol-related problems than patients who only received the standard care at the emergency room (Monti *et al.*, 1999).

There is an opposition to harm reduction strategies by some professionals that want to eliminate high risk behaviours by enforcing abstinence-only policies. This is despite widespread evidence that harm-reduction programmes can be effective and cost efficient, for example, in slowing down the spread of HIV and other communicable diseases, overdose prevention programmes, emergency room *screening* and workplace substance use prevention programmes (Marlatt and Witkiewitz, 2010).

In practice, harm reduction is most viable as an approach in health promotion when it is used in combination with other strategies, such as *peer education*, to manage high-risk behaviours.

KEY TEXTS
- Marlatt, G.A. and Witkiewitz, K. (2010) 'Update on Harm-Reduction Policy and Intervention Research', *Annual Review Clinical Psychology*, 6: pp. 591–606
- Marlatt, G.A., Larimer, M.E. and Witkiewitz, K. (2011) *Harm Reduction. Pragmatic Strategies for Managing High-Risk Behaviors*. 2nd edn (London: Guildford Press)
- Weatherburn, D. (2009) 'Dilemmas in Harm Minimization', *Addiction*, 104 (3): pp. 335–339

health activism

SEE ALSO **advocacy; boycotts; empowerment; health social movements; lobbying**

Health activism involves a challenge to the existing order whenever it is perceived to influence peoples' health negatively or has led to an injustice or an inequity (Plows, 2007).

Activism is an action on behalf of a cause, an action that goes beyond what is routine (Martin, 2007). What constitutes as activism therefore depends on what is 'conventional' in society as any action is relative to others used by individuals, groups and organizations. In practice, activist organizations employ a combination of both conventional and unconventional strategies to achieve their goals. In systems of representative government, conventional actions include election campaigning, voting, *advocacy* and *lobbying* politicians. Organizations that use these types of actions are not (and do not consider themselves as) activists because they operate using conventional means. Civil and human rights, such as the freedom of speech and expression, privacy and the right to health, are fundamental principles in many activist organizations. They are also central to the manifestos of many political parties and with whom, therefore, activist organizations are sometimes able to form an alliance (Laverack, 2013).

Activism has an explicit purpose to help to empower others and this is embodied in actions that are typically energetic, passionate, innovative and committed. It has played a major role in protecting workers from exploitation, protecting the environment, promoting equality for women and opposing racism. To some, an activist is a freedom fighter, but to others he/she is a protagonist, trouble maker, vandal or terrorist. Activism is not always used positively as the actions of some minority groups can oppose human rights and the beliefs of the majority through violent means.

The types of actions that activist organizations engage in can be broadly sub-divided into two categories: indirect and direct.

1. Indirect actions are non-violent and conventional and often require a minimum of effort, although collectively they can have a significant effect. Indirect actions include voting, signing a petition, taking part in a 'virtual (on-line) sit-in' and sending a letter or e-mail to protest your cause.
2. Direct actions can become progressively more 'unconventional', ranging from peaceful protests to inflicting intentional physical damage to persons and property. For most activists, their focus is on short term, reactive, direct tactics as their primary and often only means of action, aiming to have a real-time and immediate effect.

Direct actions can be further sub-divided into non-violent and violent actions.

2.1 Non-violent direct actions include protests, picketing, vigils, marches, rent strikes, product *boycotts*, withdrawing bank deposits, publicity campaigns and taking legal action.

2.2 Direct violent actions include physical tactics against people or property, placing oneself in a position of manufactured vulnerability to prevent action or taking part in a civil disobedience involving the damage of personal property.

Direct action can be symbolic and challenging, sending a message to the general public, and/or to the owners, shareholders, and employees of a specific company and/or to policymakers, about specific grievances and threats. Some organizations use a dual strategic approach: one that is moderate and conventional while also using unconventional and more radical tactics. The radical strategy is carried out by individuals or covert affinity groups, 'independent' of the organization, while the conventional tactics form the 'official' actions of the organization. The dynamics of this relationship are often unclear but a strategy that employs both conventional and unconventional tactics can have a significant influence on public opinion. The risk is that the unconventional tactics can result in negative publicity and impact on future resource allocation and recruitment to the organization. Some organizations do not accept donations from governments or corporations and depend instead on contributions from individuals and the assistance from volunteers in order to maintain an independent agenda. The balance between individual autonomy and group responsibility, and the relative importance of means and ends, are therefore often points of contention in using conventional and increasingly violent actions. Tactics vary from country to country and from organization to organization and the autonomy exercised by activists and their non-hierarchical structure makes a dual strategic approach both a viable and an attractive option (Martin, 2007).

The range of tactics used by activists extends from conventional, peaceful tactics to increasingly unconventional, illegal and more violent actions. If the use of conventional tactics by an organization is not successful, then it may choose to use more radical tactics as a part of the overall strategy. This is a dynamic process because organizations can use a variety of tactics, culturally informed and to some extent shaped by local laws. The tactics of health activism also continue to evolve along with political opportunity and developments in culture and technology. Cell phone messaging and the internet, for example, are now extensively used in activism to organize rallies and to carry out online tactics. Health activism is continuing to raise new issues including sexual harassment, bullying and domestic violence by campaigning about them and by developing innovative techniques to address the inequities that these issues create (Plows, 2007).

KEY TEXTS
- Andersen, G.L. and Herr, K.G. (eds) (2007) *Encyclopaedia of Activism and Social Justice* (London: Sage Publications)
- Laverack, G. (2013) *Health Activism: Foundations and Strategies* (London: Sage Publications)
- Pakulski, J. (1991) *Social Movements: The Politics of Moral Protest* (Sydney: Longman)

health and wellbeing

SEE ALSO **approaches; declarations and statements; definition; disease prevention; harm reduction; lifespan approach; lifestyle approach**

There is a multiplicity of meanings assigned to our understandings of health. In particular, it is useful to consider the distinction outlined below between official understandings, those used by health professionals, and lay understandings, the more popular perceptions held by those who are usually the recipients of health interventions.

The term 'wellbeing' is commonly used in connection with the concept of health and with the *definition* of health promotion. Wellbeing covers the social, physical and mental state and describes a satisfactory condition of existence, characterized by health, happiness and prosperity. Physical wellbeing is concerned with concepts such as the proper functioning of the body, biological normality, physical fitness and capacity to perform tasks. Social wellbeing includes interpersonal relationships as well as wider social issues such as marital satisfaction, employability and *community* involvement. The role of relations, the family and status at work are important to a person's social wellbeing. Mental wellbeing involves concepts such as self-efficacy, subjective wellbeing and social inclusion and is the ability of people to adapt to their environment and the society in which they function.

Official interpretations of health are most commonly used because these are easier to define and measure, rather than lay interpretations of health, which are subjective, being based on the experiences of the individual. In particular, the bio-medical interpretation of health has established itself as the most dominant official interpretation. It is the medical profession, which has been the champion of this approach of health, based on the absence of disease and illness, and upon which other health professions have based themselves including the field of *public health* and nursing (Laverack, 2009).

The official interpretations of health can be divided into two main types: those that define health negatively and those that adopt a more positive stance. There are two main ways of viewing health negatively. The first equates with the absence of disease or bodily abnormality, and the second with the absence of illness or the feelings of anxiety, pain or distress that may or may not accompany the disease. People may be unaware of their illness until they start to suffer pain and discomfort, when the person is said to be ill. Negative definitions of health emphasize the absence of disease or illness and are the basis for the medical approach. A number of problems have been raised concerning the negative definition of health. In particular, the notion of pathology implies that certain universal 'norms' exist against which an individual can be assessed when making a judgement as to whether or not they are healthy. This assumes that such standards actually exist in human anatomy and physiology (Aggleton, 1991).

Positive interpretations of health have also been widely used by health professionals. The first modern positive definition of health came in 1948 when the WHO stated that health was 'a state of complete physical, social and mental wellbeing, and not merely the absence of disease or infirmity' (Jackson, Mitchell and Wright, 1989). The WHO definition of health, as an ideal state of physical, social and mental wellbeing, has been criticized for not taking other dimensions of health into account, namely, the emotional and spiritual aspects of health (Ewles and Simnett, 2009). The definition has also been criticized for viewing health as an unachievable absolute and a product rather than as a dynamic relationship, a human capacity or as a potential.

The way in which people interpret the meaning of their own health is a personal and sometimes unique experience. Health is a subjective concept and its interpretation is relative to the environment and culture in which people find themselves. Health can mean different things to different people. Many people define health in functional terms by their ability to carry out certain roles and responsibilities rather than the absence of disease. People may be willing to bear the discomfort and pain of an illness because it does not outweigh the inconvenience, loss of control or financial cost of having the condition treated (Laverack, 2009). The importance of personal interpretations of health is becoming increasing well recognized, for example, the link between individual control and health. For example, Everson *et al.* (1997) undertook a study of Finnish middle-aged white males and concluded that stress induced from job demands and feelings of a lack of control was the strongest predictor of arterial heart disease.

Some commentators have concluded that it is futile to try and define health and wellbeing because it is like 'beauty' and only in the eye of the beholder. The concept of health is too complex and it is better framed within the context of the services offered and that society can afford (Jadad and O'Grady, 2008). In practice, health promotion has embraced a discourse that uses an official definition that goes beyond health care and lifestyle to feelings of wellbeing. Health is considered to be a means to an end that can be expressed in functional terms as a resource that permits people to lead an individually, socially and economically productive life. The health promotion profession has, for the time being, decide to take the pragmatic view that whatever interpretation of health is used it must be measurable and accountable; otherwise programmes employing its ideology and strategies will be in jeopardy of being unable to justify their economic and quantifiable effectiveness. This being the case, the measurement of health has focused on the bio-medical approach that is concerned with demonstrating a relationship between a health status measure and a health-related behaviour such as smoking or a condition such as mortality. The boundaries for practice and discourse have consequently been defined by the interpretations of illness and disease rather than by the way in which most people generally view or feel that they need to maintain their own health.

KEY TEXTS

- Aggleton, P. (1991) *Health* (London: Routledge)
- Ewles, L. and Simnett, I. (2009) *Promoting Health: A Practical Guide.* 5th edn, Part 1 (Edinburgh: Bailliere Tindall)
- Naidoo, J. and Wills, J. (2009) *Foundations for Health Promotion.* 3rd edn, Part 1 (Edinburgh: Bailliere and Tindall)

health communication

SEE information, education and communication

health education

SEE ALSO **behaviour change communication; definition; health literacy; information education and communication; risk factors**

While there is no universally accepted *definition* of health education, the term is traditionally regarded to represent planned opportunities for people to learn about health and to make changes to their behaviour (Naidoo and Wills, 2009, p. 58).

Health education activities include raising awareness of health issues and those *risk factors* that contribute to ill health. Awareness or consciousness raising refers to the efforts of one group of people or organization attempting to focus the attention of a wider group of people on some cause or issue such as *disease prevention*, human conflicts or political movements. It is often considered to be the first step to changing attitudes towards engagement and action. Health education provides the latest technical information, motivating people to change unhealthy behaviours and giving people the necessary skills and confidence to make those changes. Because of the nature of the activities carried out in health education, it is also associated with the concepts of *behaviour change communication, information, education and communication, health literacy* and *health communication*.

The role of the health educator is to design and implement learning activities and to provide training, instruction and skills development. The health educator is an enabler and not an 'expert' who takes an authoritarian role and tells people what they should do. The guiding principle of health education is to facilitate people to make individual informed choices about their health behaviours.

An informed choice is one that is based on relevant knowledge about a health behaviour and the perceived risk associated with a wrong choice, consistent with the decision-maker's values and behaviour (adapted from Dormandy *et al.*, 2002). The person volunteers to change their behaviour by identifying their own needs and then by taking personal actions to resolve them, such as improving their ability to perform a particular skill.

Conceptually there is still some confusion about the differences between health promotion and health education. The debate about the overlap between health promotion and health education began in the 1980s when the range of activities involved in promoting better health widened to overcome the narrow focus on lifestyle and behavioural *approaches*. These activities involved more than just giving information and aimed for strategies that achieved political action and social mobilization. The emphasis on individual responsibility had also led to accusations of 'victim blaming' that made people feel guilty about their poor state of health, even though some factors may have been outside their control, for example, being made unemployed. Tones and Tilford (2001) have suggested that health education and health promotion have a symbiotic relationship. Health education provides the agenda setting and the raising of *critical consciousness* in health promotion programmes. Without the inclusion of education strategies, health promotion programmes would be little more than manipulative processes of social coercion and *community* control. Although health education is aimed at informing people to influence their future decision making, health promotion aims at complementary social and political actions. To achieve these aims, health promotion uses strategies such as *lobbying* and community development to facilitate political changes in peoples' social, workplace and community *settings* (Green and Kreuter, 2004). Thus, health education around obesity in adolescents might include school-based awareness programmes or exercise classes. Health promotion around obesity in adolescents extends further to legislation on food advertising and restricting access to unhealthy products in school shops.

The most practical way forward in differentiating between health education and health promotion is to view the latter as encompassing the former as a range of educational and skills developing activities (Laverack, 2004).

KEY TEXTS

- Black, J.M. *et al.* (2009) *Philosophical Foundations of Health Education* (San Francisco, CA: Jossey-Bass)
- Naidoo, J. and Wills, J. (2009) *Foundations for Health Promotion*. 3rd edn (Edinburgh: Bailliere and Tindall), Chapter 4
- Tones, K. and Tilford, S. (2001) *Health Education: Effectiveness, Efficiency and Equity*. 3rd edn (Cheltenham: Nelson Thornes)

health literacy

SEE ALSO **critical consciousness; empowerment; health education; life skills**

Health literacy is a repackaging of the relationship between *health education* and *empowerment* and evolved as a concept within health promotion. Health education becomes more than just the transmission of information and is focussed on skills development and confidence so as to help others to make informed decisions that will allow them to exert greater control on their lives and health (Renkert and Nutbeam, 2001).

Health literacy grew out of the realization that interventions that relied heavily on information towards behaviour change failed to achieve substantial results and had little effect in closing the inequalities gap between different social and economic groups (Nutbeam, 2000). The unfulfilled potential of many education strategies in health promotion as a tool for social change and political action left practitioners searching for new alternatives. Health literacy involves cognitive and social skills, which determine the motivation and ability of individuals to gain access to, understand and use information in ways that promote and maintain good health (WHO, 1998).

Health literacy is dependent on the level of basic literacy in the *community*, that is, the ability to read and write in everyday life and what this enables people to do. Health literacy has three levels:

- **Basic/functional literacy:** Sufficient basic skills in reading and writing to be able to function effectively in everyday situations, broadly compatible with the narrow *definition*.
- **Communicative/interactive literacy:** more advanced cognitive and literacy skills that, together with social skills, can be used to actively participate in everyday activities, to extract

information and derive meaning from different forms of communication and to apply new information to changing circumstances.

- **Critical literacy:** more advanced cognitive skills that, together with social skills, can be applied to critically analyse information and to use this information to exert greater control over life events and situations (Nutbeam, 2000, p. 263).

The challenge in health promotion practice is to use advanced methods of health education aimed at achieving critical health literacy rather than basic or functional health literacy. The value of health literacy is as a tool to help practitioners become more effective communicators by increasing the critical awareness of individual clients.

An example of the potential use of health literacy is the development of antenatal classes to provide women with the cognitive and social skills to maintain their health and that of their children. Women attending antenatal classes are often highly motivated and literate. However, antenatal classes are sometimes constrained by time and the natural curiosity and anxiety of the women makes it difficult to transfer all the necessary information and skills. Classes, therefore, focus on the transfer of factual information rather than on decision-making skills for childbirth and parenting, which can occupy more time. The latter is empowering rather than just passive and is central to the use of health literacy techniques that focuses on providing the necessary skills and enabling women to make informed choices. In this way, the entire content of the antenatal class would not have to be delivered, reducing the time needed for teaching and providing more time to allow the mothers to ask questions and to discuss issues (Renkert and Nutbeam, 2001).

Working to raise the understanding of the underlying causes of *powerlessness* and ill health of people with poor basic literacy skills can lead to outcomes that are closely aligned with empowerment. In a health promotion practice often dominated by health education, health literacy offers an advanced strategic approach that enables people to understand better the social determinants of their health and how to take action to address them (Nutbeam, 2000).

KEY TEXTS

- Begoray, D.L., Gillis, D. and Rowlands, G. (2012) *Health Literacy in Context: International Perspectives (Public Health in the 21st Century)* (New York: Nova Science Publishers Inc)
- Nutbeam, D. (2000) 'Health Literacy as a Public Health Goal: A Challenge for Contemporary Health Education and Communication Strategies into the 21st Century', *Health Promotion International*, 15 (3): pp. 259–267
- Osborne, H. (2011) *Health Literacy: A to Z.* 2nd edn (Boston, MA: Jones and Bartlett Learning)

health policy

SEE healthy public policy

health profiles

SEE ALSO disease prevention; evaluation; healthy public policy; needs assessment

Health profiles are a summary of health information for a particular population, for example, for a country, and then further sub-divided into regions, provinces, towns and local communities (Network of Public Health Observatories, 2013).

Health profiles are used to help prioritize and plan services including health promotion. They are designed to show the differences in health (or factors that affect health) between different places, so that the right services can be put in place for each area. Health profiles need to reflect health for a diverse population throughout all stages of life and so there is a limit to the number of indicators that can be provided for any one issue. The selection of health profile indicators and content therefore requires balancing several factors including the need to highlight important *public health* topics; the need to focus on problems that can be addressed by local services; the availability of data across the entire population; the need to keep the profiles clear for users who are not familiar with medical or statistical language and the limited space available in the health profiles (Network of public health observatories, 2013).

The Estonian National Institute for Health Development (ENIHD), for example, started the process of developing health profiles in

2008, with the goal of helping communities better understand their specific health situation and determinants. The ENIHD found that as the health profiles included topics from different policy areas such as education, social services, police and urban planning, it could only be carried out with co-operation and teamwork. Communities that conducted a health profile also had an opportunity to submit project applications to the European Social Fund in Estonia. Projects had to address the solutions to problems that were evident in their health profile. In 2008, there were three *community* health profiles conducted in Estonia. By December 2012, it had reached 123 (48% of municipalities and 100% of counties). The opportunity for financial resources was a motivator, and without this, the level of community involvement in developing the health profiles would have been much lower (ENIHD, 2013).

Health impact assessment differs from a 'health profile' because it is a means of assessing the health impacts of policies, plans and projects in diverse economic sectors using quantitative, qualitative and participatory techniques. For example, transport is a major factor in traffic injuries, air pollution and noise. Healthy transport policy can help reduce these risks, as well as promoting physical activity such as walking and cycling (Taylor, Gowman and Quigley, 2003). Health impact assessment can also help *civil society* organizations to make choices about alternatives and improvements to policy, for example, the handling by authorities of the 'mad cow disease' and conflicting evidence on the benefits of *screening* for breast cancer using mammography in the United Kingdom (Smith, 2002).

Health profiles provide an indication of health in a particular population at a particular time. They are usually produced annually by the government and are made publicly available. Importantly, health profiles provide a set of important health indicators that show how one geographical area compares to the national and regional average. This comparative information then helps local government, health promotion services and civil society groups to make decisions to improve people's health and ideally to reduce health inequalities.

KEY TEXTS
- Estonian National Institute for Health Development (ENIHD) (2013) http://www.tai.ee/ [accessed 27/2/2013]

- Network of Public Health Observatories (2013) http://www.apho.org. uk/ [accessed 27/2/2013]

health protection

SEE ALSO **global health; health profiles; healthy public policy; hygiene promotion; public health**

Health protection is a term to describe activities to ensure safe food and water supplies, providing advice to national food and drug safety regulators, protecting people from environmental threats and having a regulatory framework for controlling infectious diseases (PHAC, 2013).

Ensuring proper food handling in restaurants and establishing smoke-free bylaws are examples of health-protection measures. The public image of the health-protection practitioner's role is as an enforcer of health legislation and this has been supported by the work of government departments. These services are concerned with inspection, licensing, complaint investigations and legal proceedings. An enforcement of a wide range of *public health* legislation has been seen to be necessary to maintain a healthy and safe environment, for example, at work and during recreation. Conversely, the role of the health promotion practitioner is an enabler, helper, counsellor and guide to support others to facilitate change in their lives through their own actions (Laverack, 2009).

The Health Protection Agency (HPA) is an independent UK organization that was set up by the government in 2003 to protect the public from threats to their health. The Agency is an example of how health protection brings together many of the concepts used in public health and health promotion. The Agency identifies and responds to health hazards and emergencies caused by infectious disease, hazardous chemicals, poisons or radiation. It gives advice to the public on how to stay healthy and provides data and information to government to help inform its decision making. The HPA combines public health and scientific knowledge, research and emergency planning within one organization and works at the international level to address *global health* threats. From 2013 the HPA will join Public Health England within the Department of Health to be part of the strategic *leadership* for public health, health and social care (Health Protection Agency, 2013).

Environmental health is a branch of public health that is concerned with environmental factors that affect health and overlaps with or is a term used in association with health and environmental protection. Environmental factors affecting health include, but are not limited to, air, food, water, radiation, chemicals, disease vectors, safety and housing (Friis, 2010). The political liberalism of the Victorian period in the United Kingdom, for example, led to the creation of many *pressure groups*, such as the Health of Towns Association, with a concern for equity and *social justice*. The Association promoted sanitary reform in rapidly growing areas of urban industrialization and helped key environmental health reformers, such as Edwin Chadwick, to achieve their aim of bringing in the Public Health Act 1848 and to be more active in mobilizing the middle classes who in turn had an influence on the press and on the government (Berridge, 2007). Sir Edwin Chadwick (1800–1890) was an English social reformer, noted for his work on the Poor Laws and the improvement of sanitary conditions and public health. In 1832, Chadwick was employed to inquire into the operation of and reform of the Poor. In 1834, individual parishes were formed into Poor Law Unions each with a union workhouse, although Chadwick fought for a more centralized system of administration controlled from a central board. While still officially working with the Poor Law, Chadwick also took up the question of poor sanitation. Chadwick was a commissioner of the Metropolitan Commission of Sewers in London from 1848 to 1849 and a commissioner of the General Board of Health from its establishment in 1848 to its abolition in 1854. In January 1884, he was appointed as the first president of the Association of Public Sanitary Inspectors (Chartered Institute of Environmental Health, 2012).

Today, environmental health has three basic disciplines: environmental epidemiology, toxicology and exposure science. Environmental health professionals may be known as environmental health officers, public health inspectors, sanitary inspectors or environmental specialists. Environmental health professionals are responsible for a wide range of duties including monitoring water and air quality, control of toxic substances, food hygiene inspections and ensuring safe housing targeted towards preventing disease and creating health-supportive environments (Friis, 2010).

KEY TEXTS

- Friis, R. (2010) *Essentials of Environmental Health*. 2nd edn (Boston, MA: Jones and Bartlett Learning)
- Hawker, J. *et al.* (2012) *Communicable Disease Control and Health Protection Handbook*. 3rd edn (Chichester: Wiley Blackwell)
- Health Protection Agency (UK) (2013) http://www.hpa.org.uk/. [accessed 27/2/2013]

healthy public policy

SEE ALSO **declarations and statements; definition; health activism; health profiles; health social movements**

Healthy public policy covers a range of activities and decisions that cut across a number of different sectors, for example, housing, transport and employment, and that influence quality of life, well-being and health (Baum, 2008).

Healthy public policy is one of the five key strategies in the Ottawa Charter for health promotion and is defined as 'placing health on the agenda of policy makers in all sectors and at all levels, directing them to be aware of the health consequences of their decisions and to accept their responsibilities for health' (WHO, 1986, p. 2). Healthy public policy is important to health promotion practice because it helps to change the environment in which people live and work, to enable them to make the healthy choice easier.

Healthy public policy engages with a wide range of interest groups including consumers, government services, NGOs, *pressure groups* and the commercial sector. Because of the range of issues that healthy public policy addresses, for example, drinking alcohol, smoking and reducing poverty, its formulation and development is also the target for *pressure and advocacy groups*, social movements and activists, and is intrinsically a *political activity* (Draper, 1991). The competing interests involved in many healthy public policy decisions means that its implementation will also often result in challenging the *power* of some groups that have a great deal of influence and wish to protect the interests of their shareholders, employees and members, for example, the pharmaceutical industry.

Healthy public policy can overlap with social policy as it also focuses on aspects of the economy, society and politics that are necessary to human existence, including employment, social security, housing, the promotion of health and education (Dixey *et al.*, 2013). Health policy, however, differs from healthy public policy because it is specifically concerned with the financing and operation of sickness care services. Health policy is about taking decisions, setting goals and stating ways to address them through, for example, health projects, legislation, guidelines and codes of practice (Brown, 1992).

Policy, in general, is usually made up of a combination of agendas and actions rather than just one simple decision and may be extended over a long period of time. Policy can also change over time and is influenced by many factors, including other policy decisions and stakeholders at different levels involved in the policy formulating process. Health in all policies is an approach that emphasizes that *health and wellbeing* are largely influenced by government sectors other than health and highlights the connections and interactions between different policies. A health in all policies approach is founded on health-related rights and obligations. It improves accountability of policymakers for health impacts at all levels of policy making. It includes an emphasis on the consequences of public policies on health systems, *determinants of health* and wellbeing and contributes to sustainable development. By considering health impacts across all policies such as agriculture, education, the environment, housing and transport, health outcomes can be better achieved. The health sector has an important *leadership* role to support other sectors to achieve their goals in a way that can also improves health and wellbeing (WHO, 2008). The HiAP is designed to complement a whole of government (WoG) approach, which focuses on public coherence, coordination and efficiency. More often than not, economic development is the focus of the WoG. When a health issue is not a WoG priority, then the HiAP approach can be used to engage and support other sectors to deliver the desired health and equity outcomes. If policies that serve economic goals want to improve human conditions, they must include health as an explicit policy objective.

It is sometimes difficult to define the causal links between a policy intervention and an improvement in health. The causes of many health problems are due to the social, economic and political determinants of people's lives and there can be large differences between groups, often within the same locality (Labonte and Laverack, 2008). Developing policy solutions, therefore, involves the use of a range of inter-sectoral strategies (Gauld, 2006), and sensitivity to its intrinsic political nature that should involve the communities they are designed to benefit (Yeatman, 1998). However, the people who control the political process (governments and governmental stakeholders at the national, municipal, regional and local levels) may or may not involve those who are influenced by the policy outcome. People influenced by policy decisions may not necessarily agree with this approach and may want to change its formulation or to stop its delivery. For example, the People's Health Movement (PHM) launched a campaign in 2006 to strengthen the right to health, with a focus on defending the right to health care. The campaign looks at what measures are needed to tackle human rights violations in the context of a broader analysis of power and social inequalities. It seeks social transformations indispensable to resolving such inequalities as they affect health. As such, the campaign focused on changing national and *global health* sector reform policies that affect access to health care by the poor, the disadvantaged and the marginalized. One of the key purposes of the PHM has been to give a voice to those excluded from global policy forums, and to diversify the views represented within them as a means of improving the governance of global health (Labonte and Laverack, 2008).

Several useful frameworks have been developed to conceptualize how people can act to change the 'prevailing paradigm' of policy development (Lindquist, 2001). Although they primarily reflect processes in a democratic political system, they also provide in-depth conceptualizations about how the process to influence policy development works within two broad paradigms: rationalist and political (Neilson, 2001). The rationalist paradigm includes linear, incrementalist and interactive models as representations of the policy process. It originates from classical economic theory, which presumes that actors have full information and are able to establish priorities to achieve a desired and largely uncontested goal. It is driven by the production and consideration of different forms of evidence such as public health research, as well as the input from experts and academics as a valued part of the process. The political paradigm generates policy models adapted from political economy theory and derived from comparative politics and international relations. These theories stress the importance of agenda setting, policy *networks*, policy narratives and the policy transfer in shaping final decisions. Policy decisions, in turn, are made on the basis of bargaining and negotiation between the different stakeholders who employ a range of *approaches* to have an influence on each stage of the policy process. From the vantage of policy makers, the most effective approach to policy combines elements from both the rational and political paradigms. For example, the introduction of policy to ban smoking in public places was initially based on strong epidemiological evidence regarding second-hand smoke. The best strategy to reduce death and illness from second-hand smoke would be a total ban on smoking including in homes. Obviously such a policy would be very difficult to police as well as creating opposition from civil libertarian groups. The policy decision was therefore a compromise based on the available evidence and the opposing interests of different stakeholders to reach an achievable goal rather than an optimal goal (Neilson, 2001).

KEY TEXTS
- Brown, V.A. (1992) 'Health Care Policies, Health Policies or Policies for Health?' In H. Gardner (ed), *Health Policy Development, Implementation and Evaluation in Australia* (Melbourne: Churchill Livingstone)
- Dixey, R. *et al.* (2013) *Health Promotion: Global Principles and Practice* (Wallingford, Oxfordshire: CAB International), Chapter 3
- Hunter, D. (2003) *Public Health Policy* (Cambridge, UK: Polity Press)
- Naidoo, J. and Wills, J. (2009) *Foundations for Health Promotion*. 3rd edn (Edinburgh: Bailliere and Tindall), Chapter 11

health social movements

SEE ALSO **alliances, partnerships and coalitions; empowerment; health activism; lay epidemiology; networks**

Health social movements challenge state, institutional and other forms of authority to give the public more of a voice in health policy and regulation (Brown and Zavestoski, 2004). More broadly, a social movement can be defined as a sustained and organized public effort targeting authorities that can use both conventional and unconventional strategies to achieve its goals (Tilly, 2004).

What makes a movement different from other forms of social mobilization, such as pressure and *advocacy* groups, is an ability to go beyond the influence of its participant and resource base. A social movement is able to maintain an ideology irrespective of membership, function and organizational structure. To do this, a movement must have 'deep social roots' and strong social *networks* (Laverack, 2013a). Health social movements are an important point of social interaction concerning the rights of people to access health services, personal experiences of illness, disease, disability and health inequality based on race, class, gender and sexuality. Health social movements overlap in their purpose and tactics but can be broadly categorized into three types (Brown *et al.*, 2004):

1. **Health access movements** that seek equitable access to health care services, for example, through national health care reforms and an extension of health insurance to non-insured sectors of the population.
2. **Embodied health movements** concern people who want to address personal experiences of disease, illness and disability through a challenge of the scientific evidence by medical recognition of their ideas or their own research. It can include people directly affected by a condition or those who feel they are an at risk group, for example, the HIV/AIDS movement.
3. **Constituency-based health movements** concern health inequalities when the evidence shows an oversight or disproportionate outcome, for example, the human rights movement.

The growing awareness of health science that has become available through, for example, the internet, has led to people challenging health policy. This has been coupled by the negative publicity received about, for example, experimentation with contraceptives, radiation and immunization, which has created a heightened level of distrust by the public. People have discovered that collectively they can apply significant pressure to influence policy that affects their health at both an individual and a collective level (Brown and Zavestoski, 2004).

The environmental breast cancer movement in the United States is an example of the efforts of women who were concerned with both equitable access to health care services and to addressing health inequalities. Maren Klawiter (2004) discusses the experiences of women in the 1970s in the San Francisco Bay Area with breast cancer who endured isolation and *power* inequalities structured around the doctor–patient relationship. This health social movement was created to identify with those at risk from or affected by breast cancer and provided many women with the emotional support they needed to be able to move forward collectively to address a personal issue. Using the lessons that they had brought with them they pressed for expanded clinical trials, compassionate access to new drugs and greater government funding. The health social movement used tactics such as engaging in legal action, support to new research, creative *media* campaigns and influencing the policy process (Brown and Zavestoski, 2004). Twenty years later, a new regime of breast cancer had emerged influenced by the efforts of the environmental breast cancer movement. Women had access to user-friendly cancer centres, patient education workshops, support groups, a choice of medical alternatives and a role as part of the health care team that delivered the cancer treatment. Essentially, breast cancer had become politicized and reframed as a feminist issue and an environmental disease.

The involvement in a social movement can also result in marked differences between members and non-members. For example, for those living with HIV/AIDS, members of movements had better coping skills and preferences, knowledge of HIV treatment and social network integration. The involvement in a movement had helped people to enhance their ability as individuals to make informed choices about personal health care and HIV/AIDS treatments (Brashers *et al.*, 2002).

Social movements are important to health promotion because they provide the opportunity for individuals to have greater influence by engaging in a broader participant and resource base. This then allows people to take social and political action (Labonte and Laverack, 2008) through tactics such as mass *lobbying*, protests, demonstrations and petitioning.

KEY TEXTS

- Brown, P. and Zavestoski, S. (2004) 'Social Movements in Health: An Introduction', *Sociology of Health & Illness,* 26 (6): pp. 679–694
- Staggenborg, S. (2010) *Social Movements* (Oxford: Oxford University Press)

- Tilly, C. and Lesley, J. (2012) *Social Movements, 1768–2012* (Boulder, CO: Paradigm Press)

hegemonic power

SEE ALSO **empowerment; marginalization; patient empowerment; power; powerlessness**

Hegemonic power is that form of power-over that is invisible and internalized such that it is structured into our everyday lives and taken for granted (Foucault, 1979).

To Michel Foucault, a prominent French social theorist in the twentieth century, the only form of resistance to hegemonic power was a concealment of one's life from those in authority. For example, the actions of a single mother living in poor housing to hide evidence of her drug addiction or her sick child from a health visitor (Bloor and McIntosh, 1990). Persons living in conditions of hegemonic power-over, of oppression and exploitation, internalize these conditions as being their personal responsibility. This internalization increases their own self-blame and decreases their self-esteem and can lead to a false consciousness, a failing to utilize the *power* one has and failing to acquire powers that one can acquire (Morriss, 1987). Hegemonic power is inherently unhealthy, because it shuts down critical thinking, public debate and the possibility of change. One of the subtle ways in which health practitioners participate in hegemonic power is when they continually impose their ideas of what they feel are important without listening to what others, in particular, their clients, think are important.

The rise of the medical profession has been successful in maintaining its position of dominance within the health institutional hierarchy by controlling access to health care delivery and this has been termed the 'hegemony of the medical profession'. The medical profession has successfully formed itself as a powerful professional pressure group manifested through key associations, for example, in the United Kingdom, the British Medical Association. The medical profession, although not a complete monopoly because of the growth of other health professions, has been granted considerable control to maintain self-regulation and clinical autonomy in their work. The dominance of the medical profession has, for example, been blamed for the historical subordination of the nursing profession and a key challenge to nurse *empowerment* (Kendall, 1998). Much of the power-over held by the medical profession is also supported by the public who expect confidentiality in the special relationship that they hold with their personal doctor. The medical profession is dependent on various alliances with other health professionals, the government, the private sector, science and activists in *civil society*. The medical profession has been careful to create an alignment between professional and public interests and its position further strengthened by an increase in the legitimacy of medical knowledge, urbanization, the expansion of health insurance and the growth of institutional *settings* such as hospitals as centres for 'professional excellence' (Turner and Samson, 1995).

KEY TEXTS
- Foucault, M. (1979) *Discipline and Punishment: The Birth of the Prison* (Middlesex: Penguin Books)
- Laverack, G. (2004) *Health Promotion Practice: Power and Empowerment* (London: Sage Publications), Chapter 3

hygiene promotion

SEE ALSO **disease prevention; health education; information education and communication; primary health care; public health**

Hygiene promotion is a planned approach to preventing communicable diseases, especially diarrhoeal diseases, through the widespread adoption of safe hygiene practices. Hygiene promotion encourages all the hygienic conditions and behaviours that can contribute towards good health (Appleton and Sijbesma, 2005).

Good hygiene practices are theoretically capable of reducing most instances of infection with pathogens transmitted by the faecal-oral route. In particular, simple measures, such as handwashing with soap after contact with faeces, are an acceptable intervention with large health benefits (Curtis *et al.*, 2001). Hygiene promotion starts with systematic data collection to find out and understand what different groups of people know about hygiene, what they do, what they want and why this is so. The results are used to set objectives and to identify and implement activities that enable the different groups to measurably reduce risky conditions and practices and to strengthen positive situations and behaviours.

Hygiene promotion can be delivered as a five-simple step process, as follows:

1. Action with the target communities and the team is initiated.
2. A detailed work-plan for the formative research is made.
3. The formative research is carried out.
4. An analysis and report on your results.
5. The results are fed back and discussed with key stakeholders and used to make the hygiene promotion plan (UNICEF, 1999).

PHAST is an approach based on a set of participatory techniques that has demonstrated its ability to promote hygienic behaviour, sanitation improvements and *community* management of water and sanitation facilities. PHAST is an acronym for the Participatory Hygiene and Sanitation Transformation approach and was developed in urban and rural areas in Africa. SARAR is another education and training methodology for working with stakeholders at different levels to engage their creative capacities for hygiene promotion in planning, problem solving and *evaluation*. The acronym SARAR stands for the five attributes and capacities that are considered the minimum essentials for participation to be a dynamic and self-sustaining process: self-esteem: a sense of self-worth as a person as well as a valuable resource for development; associative strength: the capacity to define and work towards a common vision through mutual respect, trust and collaborative effort; resourcefulness: the capacity to visualize new solutions to problems even against the odds, and the willingness to be challenged and take risks; action planning: combining critical thinking and creativity to come up with new, effective and reality-based plans in which each participant has a useful and fulfilling role and responsibility: for follow-through until the commitments made are fully discharged and the hoped-for benefits achieved. SARAR is based on the principle of fostering and strengthening these five attributes among the stakeholders involved in the hygiene promotion programme. SARAR enables the development of people's capacities for self-direction and management and enhances the quality of participation among all stakeholders (IRC, 2013).

An example of hygiene promotion is the 'Saniya' programme in Burkina Faso, Africa. This programme targeted the mothers and carers of young children and children of primary school age. The key messages were simply to (1) wash hands after contact with stools and (2) that stools in potties should be disposed of safely in the latrine. The programme used youth street theatre, local radio, monthly house-to-house visits, discussion groups, neighbourhood inspection teams and the development of a hygiene curriculum to channel messages to the target audience. The programme was evaluated after a three-year period and it was found that half of the mothers and carers could remember the two key messages. Hand washing after handling children's stools had increased from 13 to 31% and the number of mothers who washed their hands after using the latrine had increased by 16%. The hygiene promotion had been effective in changing behaviour because it used locally appropriate channels of communication repeated over an extended period of time. However, the popularity of hygiene promotion more evidence is needed about the costs and long-term sustained effectiveness of such programmes so as to better inform decision makers (Curtis *et al.*, 2001).

KEY TEXTS

- Appleton, B. and Sijbesma, C. (2005) *Hygiene Promotion: Thematic Overview Paper 1* (IRC International Water and Sanitation Centre, Delft, The Netherlands)
- IRC International Water and Sanitation Centre (2013) http://www.irc.nl/. [accessed 27/2/2013]
- UNICEF (1999) *A Manual on Health Promotion: Water, Environment and Sanitation Technical Guidelines. Series 6* (UNICEF: New York)

i

individualism and health

SEE ALSO healthy public policy; lifestyle approach; political activity

Individualism is an ideology that holds people responsible for their own actions and the consequences that these may have. Individualism refers to the ability of a person to make fully autonomous choices to take control of their lives and health (Tengland, 2007).

The shift in politics in westernized countries from ideologies of the left (social liberals, democrats, socialists and communists) towards the right (conservatives, capitalists and nationalists) have made individualism more influential in public policy (Baum, 2008). Government policies are promoting economic conservatism, individualism and personal responsibility for one's own life and health. This neo-liberal ideology is attractive to politicians because it (falsely) promises easily quantifiable and achievable results within a short time frame, is relatively simple (Gangolli, Duggal and Shukla, 2005) and offers powerful financial incentives for savings in health care services, especially for people suffering from chronic diseases (Bernier, 2007). Neoliberalism is a political philosophy whose advocates support economic liberalization, free trade and open markets, privatization, deregulation and decreasing the size of the public sector while increasing the role of the private sector in society (Boas and Gans-Morse, 2009).

Government health agendas typically promote individual healthy lifestyles and use motivational interventions that target the general population to change their 'unhealthy' individual behaviours. These programmes typically aim to increase awareness and develop personal skills to encourage physical activity, eating a balanced and nutritious diet, not smoking and the moderate use of alcohol. The success of these campaigns has been modest and mostly with the educated and economically advantaged in society. Subsequent improvements in health have been with higher socio-economic groups and with typically little impact on the health of the low socio-economic, ethnic minorities or indigenous people (Laverack, 2012).

The framing of health as individualized creates an obstacle because this personalization provides a focus on the 'struggle', 'fight' or 'battle' against a disease or illness. The emphasis is on self-blame, personal responsibility and individual action. Individuals may be committed to change, but this is only at the personal level and does not address the broader structural level. People who are passionate, even angry about, for example, climate change, are mobilized to protest about an issue that affects us all. However, obesity and heart disease affect us individually, and the response is to deal with these issues at a personal level. The issue is not perceived as a threat to us all and this makes collective action more difficult. However, there have been exceptions, for example, the collective action of the gay *community* in the 1980s to cope with the effects of HIV/AIDS. Such was the determination of this community that the extent of interaction was probably not seen before with regard to a health issue by both the medical profession and groups within *civil society* (Brashers *et al.*, 2002). The spread of HIV was perceived as a threat by gay men to other gay men and this motivated many of them to act collectively.

KEY TEXTS

- Baum, F. (2008) *The New Public Health*. 3rd edn (Australia and New Zealand: Oxford University Press)
- Laverack, G. (2012) 'Debate: Health Activism', *Health Promotion International*, 27 (4): pp. 429–434
- Ogden, J. (2002) *Health and the Construction of the Individual: A Social Study of Social Science* (London: Routledge)

information and communication technology

SEE ALSO **community; health social movements; media; networks**

Information and Communication Technology (ICT) is a general term for the integration of telecommunications, computers, software and audio-visuals that enables users to create, access, store, transmit and manipulate information. The term ICT is also commonly used to refer to the merging of telecommunications with computer *networks* through a single link system (Rohlinger and Brown, 2009).

ICTs allow individuals to engage with others on a broad range of social and political issues and to also provide a safe space for views to be expressed because it affords some anonymity. Online engagement through ICTs can have important implications for democratic processes, for example, in which users watch a documentary, helping to foster a local *community* and providing an opportunity for 'virtual participation' (Rohlinger and Brown, 2009). In this way, the Queer Sisters, the oldest lesbian organization in Hong Kong, has used a virtual bulletin board to create principles, ideas and feelings that challenge the status quo on homosexuality (Nip, 2004). The tactics available to health promoters via ICTs allow the sharing of contact lists for quick and easy access, permit outside agencies to link across the globe and the creation of alternative news sources. The maintenance of a website can also be an important tool for information sharing, organizing and mobilization to provide a profile and a 'face', for health promotion movements (Biddix and Han Woo, 2008).

The use of ICTs is constantly evolving and health promoters have turned to social media to engage with people online and then for activities to take place offline using networking sites, for example, the short message service (SMS). The SMS allows the interchange of text messages between mobile telephones and is the most widely used data application internationally. The capacity of the mobile telephone to organize people, record and publish images of, for example, protests, has already been established in the Middle East and in South East Asia (Banks *et al.*, 2010). Mobile telephones can also extend participation, monitoring and transparency, decentralize networks and provide opportunities for local innovation. The essential element is not high technology, but universality. Kubatana is a social and political action initiative in Zimbabwe that began on the internet, but to extend its reach adapted 'FrontlineSMS' to send out regular news updates to people who had either no news source at all or none that was trustworthy. It was soon discovered that the system was valued for its capacity to operate as a genuine information exchange, putting people from across the country in touch with one another (Banks *et al.*, 2010).

The world-wide web is an important source of specific health information, for example, a survey of over 500 users who went online for health care information found that 93% were looking for a specific illness or condition and 65% were looking for information about nutrition, exercise or weight control (Fox and Rainie, 2001). Another survey of 1,700 patients in the United Kingdom accessing a health information website showed a high patient demand for online health services such as booking GP appointments and ordering repeat medication. Almost half of the respondents (47%) were aged over 55, indicating that demand for internet-based health services is not limited to younger patients and that over three quarters of respondents (78%) were female (Patient UK, 2012).

In a rapidly changing *media* environment, health promoters have to continue to take advantage of the world-wide web, the internet and other forms of social media such as facebook, twitter and Youtube, to better communicate, organize, mobilize, lever and raise resources for their respective causes.

KEY TEXTS
- Banks, K. *et al.* (2010) *SMS Uprising: Mobile Activism in Africa* (Oxford: Fahamu Books and Pambazuka Press)
- Glaser, J. and Salzberg, C. (2011) *The Strategic Application of Information Technology in Health Care Organisations* (San Francisco, CA: Jossey Bass)
- Noar, S.M. and Grant-Harrington, N. (2012) *eHealth Applications: Promising Strategies for Behaviour Change* (New York: Routledge)

information, education and communication

SEE ALSO **counselling and one-to-one communication; critical consciousness; health education; information and communication technologies**

Information, education and communication (IEC) is an approach that is based on the need to make all concerned more effective communicators by using a mix of appropriate channels (Hubley, Copeman and Woodall, 2013).

IEC not only emerged from family planning activities in the 1970s and 1980s in westernized countries but has also been used to promote a variety of issues including hygiene and child rights. Different forms of communication used in IEC include the mass media, face to face, traditional forms of entertainment and the internet. These *approaches* are used to reach a large audience rapidly and at a relatively low cost. Print media include posters, leaflets, booklets and flip charts and can be used as a part of one-to-one communication to assist the transfer of information and skills when working with both literate and non-literate populations. The visual images are used to generate a two-way discussion between the practitioner and their clients and is especially useful in a teaching environment such as with school children using participatory techniques.

Communication strategies have traditionally been implemented using only one or two channels, for example, a mass media campaign on road safety. This is because the frequency and design of communication activities has often been determined by the availability of resources. A simple approach that combines different communication channels as a part of the same intervention can make IEC more effective. Each communication channel is used to reinforce the same key messages and are implemented on a regular basis as part of the intervention, for example, weekly radio broadcasts, the distribution of leaflets and counselling sessions. An 'opportunistic channel' is also included, such as *community* theatre, one that is used when the opportunity arises, usually when people congregate in a public place, for example, at clinics, in shopping malls or leisure centres. The combination of channels are designed to be used together to strengthen the approach, for example, formal didactic methods can be made more participatory when used with teaching aids such as flipcharts. It is important that the target audience(s) is clearly identified and that the message content is specific and consistently delivered through the different channels of communication. The materials must be attractive in design, well presented, clear and entertaining to appeal to the target audiences. The approach should be low cost so that production and distribution can be reasonably sustained, for example, by using low-cost leaflets for clients to read at home.

Other terms such as health communication are sometimes used to include IEC. *Health communication* is a key strategy to inform the public about health concerns and to maintain important health issues on the public agenda. The purpose of health communication is to improve the health status of individuals and populations. The use of the mass and multi-media and other technological innovations to disseminate health information to the public increases awareness of specific aspects of individual and collective health. Health communication, such as IEC, encompasses several areas including edutainment or enter-education, health journalism, interpersonal communication, media advocacy, organizational communication, risk communication and *social marketing*. It can also take many forms from mass and multi-media communications to traditional and culture-specific communication such as storytelling, puppet shows and songs (Communication, Education and Participation, 1996).

IEC helps people to gain more control over their lives and health by providing an increase in health knowledge and skills, for example, for the preparation of an oral rehydration solution. Information also helps them to make a specific 'informed choice or decision' to have greater control with regard to health, for example, the benefits of breast feeding or immunization. An increase in the understanding of the underlying causes of their lack of *power*, for example, unemployment and a low income enables them to take the necessary action to improve their circumstances (Laverack, 2009).

KEY TEXTS

- Laverack, G. and Dao, H.D. (2003) 'Transforming Information, Education and Communication in Vietnam', *Health Education*, 103 (6): pp. 363–369
- Schiavo, R. (2007) *Health Communication: From Theory to Practice* (San Francisco, CA: Jossey-Bass)
- Wright, K., Sparks, L. and O'Hair, D. (2012) *Health Communication in the 21st Century*. 2nd edn (London: Wiley Blackwell)

injury prevention

SEE ALSO **disease prevention; harm reduction; lifestyle approach**

Injury prevention is an effort to prevent or reduce the severity of bodily injuries caused by external mechanisms, before they occur, to improve the health of the population (Pless and Hagel, 2005).

Injury is a leading cause of death and disability including most significantly, from road traffic injuries. Injuries have two main divisions: intentional and unintentional. Intentional injury includes homicide in all forms: war, violence, terrorism, abuse and suicide.

Unintentional includes all other forms of injury. However, there can be some overlap between the two divisions, for example, when risky behaviour leads to injury such as in extreme sports. Injury prevention interventions include safety measures for boats and the water, consumer products, firearms, in the home, occupational and children and cover a variety of *approaches*, many of which are classified as falling under the '6Es'. The 6Es of injury prevention are education, engineering, enforcement, *evaluation*, economic incentives and *empowerment*. Injury prevention is seen as being a preferable term to accident prevention. The reasoning is that the common meaning attached to the word 'accident' is a random or chance event, and thus one that cannot be prevented. Most injuries, on the other hand, are predictable and therefore preventable (Baker *et al.*, 1991).

Primary injury prevention applies to the prevention of the initial event, but in many instances this is not possible. To the extent to which such events are predictable, it is often the case that the only strategy that is conceivable, but rarely feasible and often undesirable, is to reduce or eliminate exposure to risk. Secondary prevention interventions happen after an injury has occurred. The goal is to limit long-term disability and prevent re-injury, for example, providing suitably modified working conditions for injured workers. Tertiary injury prevention reduces or eliminates long-term impairment and disabilities, minimize suffering and might include rehabilitation. The focus is not on preventing the injury but its consequences, for example, prompt transfer to minimize brain damage after head trauma (Pless and Hagel, 2005).

An example of one injury prevention intervention in the United States was carried out over a six-year period in nursing homes, covering 552 licensed beds. On the basis of a 'best practice' approach, the purpose of the intervention was to reduce back injury in 1728 nursing employees. The key elements of the intervention were the use of mechanical lifting and repositioning equipment, the training of nursing personnel in the correct use of the equipment and a 'zero lift' policy assessing each residents' lifting needs and procedures for safe handling. The training was modified to provide instruction to two nurses at a time so as best to demonstrate how the equipment should be operated. An evaluation of the intervention found that these simple measures significantly reduced the rate, severity and cost of injuries. The number of lost and restricted work days was also significantly reduced. An additional benefit was that the number of assaults by residents towards nursing staff also declined during lifting and repositioning (Collins *et al.*, 2004).

KEY TEXTS

- Baker, S. *et al.* (1991) *The Injury Fact Book* (New York: Oxford University Press)
- Christoffel, T. and Gallagher, S. (2005) *Injury Prevention and Public Health: Practical Knowledge, Skills and Strategies* (Boston, MA: Jones and Bartlett Learning)
- Pless, B. and Hagel, B. (2005) 'Injury Prevention: A Glossary of Terms', *Journal of Epidemiology and Community Health,* 59 (3): pp. 182–185

1

lay epidemiology

SEE ALSO empowerment; health profiles; healthy public policy; individualism and health

Lay epidemiology describes the processes by which people in their everyday life understand and interpret risks (Allmark and Tod, 2006), including risks to their *health and wellbeing*.

To reach conclusions about risks, people access information from a variety of sources including the mass media, the internet, friends and family. For example, in India, the People's Health Movement has conducted a number of people's tribunals where evidence of the lack of access to health care and its damaging effects have combined with court actions to hold the government accountable to its domestic and international legal obligations to maintain health services (Peoples Health Movement, 2012).

Lay epidemiology can be an empowering experience for ordinary people and can help them to challenge the accepted 'wisdom' of health professionals in the following ways:

1. People through reaching their conclusions do not necessarily accept health messages. People have recognized that some health messages are 'half-truths' that can also change, for example, with regard to safe limits for alcohol consumption. Practitioners have chosen to use simple messaging that does not tell the whole truth by exaggerating the risks of a particular behaviour or the benefits of changing that behaviour. The *prevention paradox* is that targeting the behaviour of the majority who are at a low-to-medium risk has little effect at the individual level. For example, reducing dietary fat consumption for the whole population would reduce coronary heart disease, but it is difficult to change the behaviour of those whose risk is only low to medium. However, an over reliance on *health education approaches* has led to mistrust in the public, people

feel that risk does not apply to them and they reject the advice (Hunt and Emslie, 2001).

2. People have cultural and personal values that undermine the meaning of health messages, for example, a person can choose not to give up smoking simply because it may be damaging to their health when they believe that the benefits of smoking, such as for pleasure or to reduce stress, outweigh the risk.

3. People can view any particular health behaviour in at least three ways: (1) It is bad because it is poisonous. (2) It is bad but desirable such as smoking. (3) It is bad in some ways but good in others such as consuming alcohol. People's perception of risk therefore depends on their circumstances, culture and values and an 'all things considered' approach is taken (Allmark and Tod, 2006).

Communities are influenced by the information that they receive, sometimes from many conflicting sources, and that they feel can place them at risk. For example, in the United Kingdom, public concerns were raised about the Measles, Mumps and Rubella vaccine. The public health authorities saw this as an effective option with few side effects. However, following *media* reports of conflicting scientific evidence, the public became increasingly concerned that the vaccine could lead to bowel cancer and autism (Smith, 2002) and refused to have their children immunized.

In contrast to lay epidemiology, social epidemiology provides a measure of the wellbeing of populations, documenting and establishing trends based on its 'expert' and 'legitimate' *power*. Social epidemiology is the systematic study of health, wellbeing, social conditions or problems and diseases and their determinants, using epidemiology and social science methods to develop interventions, programmes and policies that can lead to a reduction in any adverse impact on populations (Cwikel, 2006). Social epidemiology emphasizes that it is the study, by qualified researchers, of social problems in combination with epidemiology linked to the heath status of populations. This sets standards of 'normality' that can be compared with relation to other population groups. In this way, health practice can build upon political concerns and create issues that they show can be overcome by using their 'expert' knowledge and power. The public is open to rational discussion and practitioners can engage with communities to offer advice that is based on sound scientific evidence. Health experts can play a mediating role between those in authority and those in *civil society* by helping to shape their daily conduct through rationality, research and self-regulation.

Lay epidemiology poses a challenge to those in authority in the health sector because it does not accept the professional 'wisdom', which then is no longer the dominant perspective. Of course, the means of governing people is also dependant on 'expert' systems of knowledge, science and empirical truths. This is a means to regulate how practitioners are empowered to control health care, knowledge and a variety of social problems that do not necessarily fall within the bio-medical sphere. The authority structures with regard to health are part of the power-over that the state has on society (Brown and Zavestoski, 2004). However, attempts to coerce or manipulate the public can place lay epidemiology as a means for their dissatisfaction to be validated and as a means to *empowerment*.

KEY TEXTS
- Allmark, P. and Tod, A. (2006) 'How Should Public Health Professionals Engage with Lay Epidemiology?' *Journal of Medical Ethics,* 32: pp. 460–463
- Cwikel, J.G. (2006) *Social Epidemiology: Strategies for Public Health Activism* (New York: Columbia University Press)
- Oakes, M. and Kaufman, J. (2006) *Methods in Social Epidemiology* (San Francisco, CA: Jossey Bass)

leadership

SEE ALSO **alliances, partnerships and coalitions; competencies; declarations and statements; gender and health; health activism; leverage**

Leadership can be described as a process of social influence in which one person can enlist the aid and support of others in the accomplishment of a shared task and is often seen as somebody whom people follow, who guides or directs others (Chemers, 1997).

For many years, the WHO has provided the global direction and leadership that has helped to shape the way we view health promotion today. This has been marked by key international conferences, documents and charters including the Ottawa Charter for Health

Promotion (WHO, 1986) and the Bangkok Charter for Health Promotion in a Globalized World (WHO, 2005). The WHO has had a significant role in orchestrating these milestones through its international convening powers. However, the relevance of the WHO, its future within *global health* governance and its own organizational crisis has raised the question: Where are the individuals and organizations that can provide the global leadership and vision for health promotion in the future? A leadership style that can work with the many actors and *approaches* in health promotion and yet maintain the international profile necessary to *leverage* its cross-sectoral role is necessary. This might be best represented as a consortium of individual leaders or a lead organization that hold the qualities of good leadership (Laverack, 2012a).

The qualities of good leadership at an individual or organizational level include being charismatic, visionary, passionate, reflective and politically savvy. Alternatively, typologies of competency, the ways in which a leader puts into practice traits in order to influence other people, place an emphasis on motivating, inspiring, collaborating, communicating and empowering. Typologies, whether of characteristics, *competencies*, situational variables or styles, share the notion that leadership is divisible into observable components. The leadership relationship with other members of the group is especially important and the leader is not in isolation but is in an interaction with his/her followers. Good leaders are aware of the efforts of the members of the organization who, behind the scenes, strive tirelessly doing day-to-day and often mundane activities. Good communication and self-reflection skills are also key elements and leaders have to be creative and able to adapt to challenges of rapid change (Frusciante, 2007).

Health promotion leaders act as figureheads, spokespeople, role models, strategists, visionaries and intellectuals within the profession. However, once charismatic leaders have gone, their vision may not be continued and internal conflict means that the organization loses its impetus. Mechanisms must exist to ensure the continuity of vision even after leaders have left. A solution to the problem is selecting a mix of different types of leaders or else making a conscious commitment to sharing *power* and an opposition to formal hierarchy. Such groups might adopt consensus decision making and encourage everyone to develop a range of skills and play a variety of roles in the organization. Leadership still exists in such groups, but it is leadership based on contributions and respect, not formal roles (Martin, 2007).

The range of skills that health promotion require includes encouraging and supporting the ideas and planning efforts of others, using democratic decision-making processes and the sharing of information. The ability to boost the confidence of participants and develop in them a belief that they can succeed, to promote teamwork and to motivate those around them. Another important skill is in *conflict resolution, advocacy* and the ability to connect to other leaders and organizations to gain resources and establish partnerships (Kumpfer, 1995).

Leaders who have a commitment to public involvement are also important to motivate others and to develop partnerships. In one organization local people were drawn into the process of participation and with increased confidence and capacity became powerful advocates in their own *community*. A proper balance between leadership and lay people was seen as essential because conflict was found to occur when there as a lack of clarity of who had decision-making influence (Anderson, Shepard and Salisbury, 2006).

Leaders do not necessarily have the skills to motivate and organize people and may lack the experience needed in their role as a manager. Good leadership therefore involves both personal and organizational qualities and characteristics such as a decision-making style, networking and political efficacy. Leaders need to take responsibility for getting things done, dealing with conflict and providing a clear direction. In simple terms, an effective leader must be a good manager and an organizer, the person who decides what needs to be done and then gets people to do it. Leadership and management is an iterative process in which people learn by doing, reflecting on the outcomes, learning from mistakes and by putting these lessons into practice. Effective leaders also manage time properly, foster a commitment at an early stage and maintain ongoing involvement of all the members of the organization in the cause. In particular, a steering group, task force or committee can be a useful way to keep the direction of the organization on track. The qualities of a successful steering committee are of people who are prepared to put time and skills into the process at strategic levels. The committee provides regular feedback to the members and an opportunity to reflect and act on the lessons learnt and to follow-up on recommendations (Smithies and Webster, 1998).

Change can be a threatening process, but new ideas and innovations, which may be necessary for the growth or survival of the organization, are more likely to be accepted if they come from within the organization rather than from an outside source. Autocratic management techniques can create a lack of trust between the leadership and the members of the organization. The involvement of the members of the organization by the leadership is therefore an essential part of introducing and adapting to change (Hubley, Copeman and Woodall, 2013).

KEY TEXTS
- Hubley, J., Copeman, J. and Woodall, J. (2013) *Practical Health Promotion*. 2nd edn (Cambridge, UK: Polity Press)
- Johnson, J. and Breckon, D. (2006) *Managing Health Education and Promotion Programs: Leadership Skills for the 21st Century*. 2nd edn (Boston, MA: Jones and Barlett Publishers)
- Rowitz, L. (2013) *Public Health Leadership*. 3rd edn (Boston, MA: Jones and Bartlett Learning)

leverage

SEE ALSO **boycotts; community capacity building; empowerment; lobbying; political activity; power; powerlessness; zero and non-zero-sum**

Leverage occurs when people bring more varied experience, widespread contacts and a longer track record than others, and this additional input can be seen as advantageous to lever or gain greater influence. More specifically, leverage refers to the ability to influence people or events to get things done (Rathgeber, 2009).

Leverage may be achieved through the application of funds to attract further financial support from others or it may refer to the participation of others in achieving goals. In essence, individuals or organizations use their assets, including their knowledge, expertise, past achievements and funds, as a 'lever' to help gain a greater political influence and to have a pivotal role both within their own context and in the broader arena. To achieve a pivotal role, it is not always necessary to reach a critical mass of people, but merely for individuals within the group to see themselves as part of the collective and to identify strategic pathways to influence health policy making and resource allocation. However, resources are seldom sufficient (even in higher income countries) and there are many competing interests. Consequently, the 'leveraging' that is carried out will have to include a political component to convince decision makers, who have control over resources, to invest in a particular issue and to listen to the knowledge, skills and expertise of local people (Rathgeber, 2009).

Leverage is therefore used to raise the position of a person or group, while simultaneously lowering it for another person or group. Leverage is a form of *zero-sum power* in which one can only possess x amount of power to the extent that someone else has the absence of an equivalent amount. My power-over you, plus your absence of that power, equals zero (thus the term, 'zero-sum'). I win and you lose. For you to gain power, you must seize it from me. If you can, you win and I lose (Laverack, 2004).

Leverage strategies differ according to circumstances and include *advocacy*, protests, *lobbying, boycotts* and petitions, but the objective remains the same: to add to the level of influence that an individual, a group or an organization has by harnessing additional assets (Laverack, 2013).

An example of the use of leverage is by the anti-sweatshop movement. Large garment corporations are vulnerable targets for anti-sweatshop action because their buyer-driven character forces them to survive in highly competitive markets. To make a profit, they must compete with other sellers over consumers looking for good-quality clothing at very affordable prices. To maintain and even improve their market shares and profit margins, they outsource their manufacturing to countries where labour is inexpensive and devote resources to marketing. In the weakly regulated setting of outsourced garment manufacturing, worker welfare is jeopardized by the fast and flexible production needed to keep up with fashion. The anti-sweatshop movement has used the vulnerable and competitive situation of the buyer-driven corporate world to lever for an improvement in garment workers' rights. Wanting profits and a good image among consumers, logo garment corporations are now being forced to address sweatshop problems (Micheletti and Stolle, 2007).

Leverage can be used in health promotion programmes as part of capacity-building *approaches* to help facilitate more varied experience through networking, knowledge and skills through training or finances through resource mobilization. The purpose is to create a more advantageous situation for the participants of the programme (individuals, groups and communities) to lever or gain greater influence.

KEY TEXTS
- Laverack, G. (2013) *Health Activism: Foundations and Strategies* (London: Sage Publications), Chapter 8
- Naidoo, J. and Wills, J. (2009) *Foundations for Health Promotion*. 3rd edn (Edinburgh: Bailliere and Tindall), Chapter 7

life skills

SEE ALSO **critical consciousness; health literacy; lifespan approach; peer education; self-help groups**

Life skills are abilities for adaptive and positive behaviour that enable individuals to deal effectively with the demands and challenges of everyday life. Life skills consist of personal, inter-personal, cognitive and physical skills, which enable people to control and direct their lives and to develop the capacity to live with and produce change in their environment (WHO, 1998, p. 15).

Life or personal skills for health promotion are described as one of the key action areas in the Ottawa Charter that states 'health promotion supports personal and social development through providing information, education for health, and enhancing life skills' (WHO, 1986, p. 3). By so doing, it increases the options available to people to exercise more control over their own health and over their environments, and to make choices conducive to health. Enabling people to learn, throughout life, to prepare themselves for all of its stages and to cope with chronic illness and injuries is essential. This is facilitated in school, home, work and *community settings* through educational, professional, commercial and voluntary bodies, and within the institutions themselves (WHO, 1986).

Examples of individual life skills include decision making and problem solving, creative and critical thinking, self-awareness and empathy, communication skills and interpersonal relationship skills and coping with emotions. In practice, these translate into everyday health skills such as smoking cessation, breastfeeding, hand-washing, coping with stress and bullying. *Health literacy*, for example, has been specifically developed within health promotion to allow the practitioner to focus on the skills and confidence development of their clients so as to exert greater control on their lives and health.

The contemporary models of health promotion have advanced to use a holistic approach of the Ottawa Charter that identify upstream socio-economic variables such as poverty, equity, *social justice* and *empowerment*. The terms upstream and downstream refer to the level of intervention, in this case in health promotion, to positively impact on the health of people. At the individual (downstream) level, people may be treated for a condition based on targeted strategies such as *screening* for early signs of disease such as breast screening. At the population (upstream) level, health promotion works to address the *determinants of health* that relate to the conditions under which people live. The terms originate from Zola's analogy of busily dragging drowning people from a flooded river (downstream) without going (upstream) to discover the reason and prevent those people from falling or being pushed into the river. Downstream interventions are sometimes considered to be futile and short term and that the focus of health promotion should be addressing the structural causes of poverty and *powerlessness* that create poor health in the first instance (McKinlay, 1979). The resulting upstream causality thinking has yielded a complex contemporary discussion of attribution of effect that embraces the social determinants of health with a greatly diminished regard to personal skills that are seen as individual-based traditional *health education* (McQueen and De Salazar, 2011).

KEY TEXTS

- McQueen, D. and de Salazar, L. (2011) 'Health Promotion, the Ottawa Charter and "Developing Personal Skills": A Compact History of 25 Years', *Health Promotion International*, 26 (Supplement 2): pp. 194–201
- Nutbeam, D. (2000) 'Health Literacy as a Public Health Goal: A Challenge for Contemporary Health Education and Communication Strategies into the 21st Century', *Health Promotion International*, 15 (3): pp. 259–267

- World Health Organization (1986) *Ottawa Charter for Health Promotion* (Geneva: World Health Organization)

lifespan approach

SEE ALSO empowerment; life skills; lifestyle approach; theories and models

The lifespan approach to health promotion focuses on how our needs and bodies change throughout our lives. The approach is based on providing appropriate interventions at the different stages of a person's lifespan to promote *health and wellbeing* (Hubley, Copeman and Woodall, 2013).

Lifespan can be described in many ways such as biological, educational, economic, social and cultural stages. However, age in years is most often used, although this can create some overlap between the different stages in health promotion interventions.

When planning a health promotion lifespan approach, it is therefore important to carefully identify which age groups the intervention will focus on and this, in part, will also be determined by the demographics of the target population. Within the specific age groups that have been selected, it is then necessary to identify the health promotion needs and strategies that can be most effectively used. This is because people are faced with different *risk factors* and have access to different communication stages in their lifespan. A basic lifespan framework for health promotion would typically use the following stages: pre-conception to birth; pre-school (0–4 years); pre-pubescent school age (5–9 years); pubescent and adolescent (10–17 years); young person (18–24 years); middle adult (25–49 years); older adult (50–69 years) and elderly (70+).

- From pre-conception to birth, the health of the baby is affected by the nutrition and health of the mother. Health promotion interventions would include policy promotion for folic acid to reduce the risk of spina bifida and education programmes to ensure that the mother did not drink alcohol or smoke and had a balanced diet. *Health literacy* and *life skills* interventions would also be used for the ante and prenatal periods to safeguard both the mother and child including promoting breastfeeding.
- The first years of life are a period of rapid physical and psychological development and health promotion interventions

such as promoting social and mental stimulation, nutrition and support to parents are important.

- The pre-pubescent school age child is exposed to a much wider circle of contacts and who may be subject to bullying and abuse. Health promotion interventions for this age are most often channelled through the school setting as well as through social clubs and interest groups.
- The pubescent and adolescent school age marks major physical changes as well as a social dimension in which there is a transition from childhood to adulthood. Health promotion interventions also change and begin to place more responsibility on the individual for their own behaviour related to, for example, substance abuse, pregnancy and sexually transmitted diseases. A key consideration when working with adolescents is at what age they begin to understand the social world in a concrete and abstract way such that they can fully engage with concepts of a political nature. An approach to adolescence based on rights, or the participation agenda, sees them as social actors who act on the world around them. Practitioners can then engage with them about their worlds and involve them in decision making. Although there is not a definitive 'youngest' age at which adolescents can be engaged to empower themselves collectively, my own inquiries into this issue have led to a guide of 14 years, give or take a year, depending on the individual (Laverack, 2013). Schools are seen as an important setting for health promotion because they can be used to reach a large audience for a long period of time. The learning of health-related knowledge, attitudes and behaviours begin at an early, school age. The development of school *health education*, for example, also reflects the development of health promotion. Sex education in schools is now called 'sex and relationships' in an attempt to move away from a medial model focus on biology to a focus on broader emotional, values and life skills necessary for adolescents to deal with this issue in their lives (Naidoo and Wills, 2009).
- In many cultures, a young person legally and socially becomes an adult at the age of approximately 18 years. However, it is also a confusing time in which many pressures are placed on the young person, such as employment or continued education,

and can lead to tension and conflict in their lives. Health promotion interventions may target substance abuse, isolation and mental illnesses through, for example, *peer education* and social media.

- Middle adulthood is a time for establishing a pattern in life, raising a family and breaking relationships. The role of health promotion is to ensure that people are supported on a range of health and parenting issues often through a range of services such as clinical *settings*, health workers and child-care services.
- Older adulthood is the start of a transition to being elderly and a period when people can suffer from chronic diseases such as cancers and heart disease. The emphasis is on maintaining a healthy lifestyle and coping with life changing experiences such as bereavements and the menopause.
- It is important to distinguish between the 'well old' and the 'frail old' as it is in the latter that the elderly person will need special attention from health promotion interventions. Key concerns are isolation, disability, osteoporosis, abuse and coping with poverty such as keeping warm in winter and having a balanced diet (Hubley, Copeman and Woodall, 2013).

KEY TEXTS

- Beckmann Murray, R., Proctor Zentner, J. and Yakimo, R. (2009) *Health Promotion Strategies through the Life Span*. 8th edn (New Jersey: Pearson Education Inc)
- Edelman, C. and Mandle, C. (2009) *Health Promotion throughout the Life Span*. 7th edn (New York: Elsevier/Mosby Publishers)
- Hubley, J., Copeman, J. and Woodall, J. (2013) *Practical Health Promotion*. 2nd edn (Cambridge, UK: Polity Press)

lifestyle approach

SEE ALSO **approaches; determinants of health; individualism and health; lifespan approach; theory and models**

A lifestyle approach is a way of living based on identifiable patterns of behaviour that are determined by the interplay between an individual's personal characteristics, social interactions and socioeconomic and environmental living conditions (WHO, 1998, p. 16).

At the time of its publication, the Lalonde report (1974) had a considerable influence on *health education* thinking. The report used the 'health field' approach that argued health was determined more by biology, genetics, the environment and human behaviour than by the provision of health services. The term 'lifestyle' entered the discourse as a total of behaviours that made up the way people lived, worked and played.

However, individual lifestyles, characterized by identifiable patterns of behaviour, also have a profound effect on an individual's health and on the health of others. If *health* is to be improved by enabling individuals to change their lifestyles, action must be directed not only at the individual but also at social and living conditions that interact to produce and maintain these patterns of behaviour. It is important to recognize, however, that there is no optimal lifestyle to be prescribed for all people. Culture, income, family structure, age, physical ability, home and the work environment will make certain ways and conditions of living more attractive, feasible and appropriate (WHO, 1998, p. 16).

The lifestyle approach became increasingly central to health promotion in the 1970s when health promoters (though many still called themselves health educators) recognized that individuals' behaviours and lifestyle could directly influence their own health and the health of others. The strategies used in the lifestyle approach were the education and awareness raising of individuals to allow them to make 'informed choices' about their lifestyle and to avoid 'high-risk' behaviours. This worked on the assumption that changing knowledge would also lead to a change in a person's attitude and practice, for example, with regard to smoking cessation. This was found to be overly simplistic and with an emphasis on individual responsibility, which did not address external forces, led to 'victim blaming'. Health is individualized by people who regard it as personal in nature and there can be a tendency to blame them for their ill health, as people are responsible for the things, both good and bad, that happen to them. Other theories to explain behaviour change focusing on the individual became more widely used including the Health Belief Model, the social learning theory and the trans-theoretical (stages of change) approach (Nutbeam, Harris and Wise, 2010). As the lifestyle approach developed, it began to recognize that behaviour is not an isolated action under the autonomous control of the individual, but that it is influenced and conditioned by a complex interplay of social, political and cultural factors. Much of health promotion work continues to use the lifestyle approach, with a focus on the individual rather than on their broader socio-economic context and the *determinants of health*.

Two well-known lifestyle *approaches* in the United States were the Multiple Risk Factors Intervention Trial (MRFIT) and the Community Intervention Trials for Smoking Cessation (COMMIT). The MRFIT was a ten-year programme designed to reduce mortality from heart disease in the top 10 per cent male risk group. The trial undertook a massive survey of 400,000 men in 22 cities and randomly selected 6,000 for the intervention and 6,000 for the control group. The trial was the most ambitious, expensive and intensive anywhere tried at the time in 1971. The trial failed and after six years the men in the intervention group did not achieve a lower mortality level from coronary heart disease than men in the control group. The COMMIT consisted of nationwide studies involving over 10,000 heavy smokers in 11 cities with a matched control group. At the end of this trial, there was only a modest difference in the rate of people stopping smoking between the intervention and control groups. The trial, which cost millions of dollars and used a team of highly motivated and trained 'experts' to implement, similarly failed (Syme, 1997).

An analysis of the small degree of success of lifestyle programmes identified that motivation to change behaviour must come from the person and cannot come from an expert. However, accepting the expertise of lay health knowledge, and sharing professional expertise so that community members can use it to build their own empowering capacities, is alien to many health professionals.

Providing education and awareness activities to influence individual behaviour does play a role in health promotion, but this must support the underlying social, economic and political issues that have been identified as being relevant and important to also have an influence on the broader context in which people live (Syme, 1997).

KEY TEXTS
- Kohl III, H. and Murray, T. (2012) *Foundations of Physical Activity and Public Health* (Illinois: Human Kinetics)

- Naidoo, J. and Wills, J. (2009) *Foundations for Health Promotion.* 3rd edn (Edinburgh: Bailliere and Tindall)
- Nutbeam, D., Harris, E. and Wise, M. (2010) *Theory in a Nutshell. A Practical Guide to Health Promotion Theories.* 3rd edn (London: McGraw-Hill)

lobbying

SEE ALSO **advocacy; boycotts; leverage; political activity**

Lobbying is an attempt to influence official decisions through the direct and personal communication between a lobbyist and the policymaker (McGrath, 2007a).

Lobbying has been criticized on the grounds that it affords undue influence over public policy to powerful and resourced interests at the expense of those groups that are already less favoured. Its defenders assert that lobbying is merely the manifestation by a group of its freedom of expression and a mechanism by which people are able to communicate directly with elected representatives. The term 'lobbying' probably originates from Members of Parliament in the United Kingdom who could be met by their constituents and others in the Central Lobby of the House of Commons in the nineteenth century. Lobbying is a feature of the policy-making process in every democratic system and lobbyists commonly describe themselves as forming a bridge between government and the governed, across which information can flow in order to ensure that policy decisions are better informed and that people can interact with policymakers more frequently. Policy makers also find it useful to be provided with information by lobbyists about the possible impact of a policy decision. Much lobbying involves a relatively straightforward supply of information, often in the interests of the group providing it. If a policy maker hears from the range of groups lobbying on an issue, they will be better informed about the issue and thus better able to reach a position on it. This should not imply, however, that lobbying is a wholly unrestricted activity. Professional lobbyists in some countries, such as the United States, must register with Congress and must provide information on their activities and expenditures. Most lobbying is directed at those policy makers who already favour a group's interests or at those who have not yet arrived at a firm view on an issue, rather than being aimed at persuading a policy maker to radically change his or her mind (McGrath, 2007a).

Grassroots lobbying is based on the idea that 'all politics is local' and that the more constituents who write or call about an issue, the more likely their elected representatives are to pay attention to it. Grassroots lobbying campaigns in which politicians are contacted by large numbers of voters, expressing a strong desire for the politician to support or oppose a policy proposal, can give politicians a signal as to how significant a policy decision may be (Laverack, 2013). Crucial to the effectiveness of a grassroots lobbying effort, though, is not so much the number of constituent communications generated, but rather that all communications demonstrate the individual voter's genuine views and, as much as possible, relate those views to the constituent's situation. Not In My Backyard (NIMBY) and the term 'Nimbyism' are used to describe the opposition by people, often local residents, to a proposal for a new development such as an industrial park, wind farm, landfill site, road, railway line or airport in their neighbourhood. NIMBY often starts grassroots lobbying campaigns when group supporters write, phone, fax, or e-mail their elected officials to express a view about a given forthcoming policy decision (Hull, 1988). Another popular technique is a 'Lobby Day' involving people converging on the office of their local political representative to meet them in an organized way to deliver their message in order to signal a strong commitment to the issue. A variant of grassroots campaigns is referred to as 'grasstops' efforts, in which a group attempts to identify and activate a smaller number of particularly influential individuals. These may be the friends, former colleagues, neighbours of the politician or key local opinion formers such as business or religious leaders (McGrath, 2007).

KEY TEXTS

- Laverack, G. (2013) *Health Activism: Foundations and Strategies* (London: Sage Publications), Chapter 8
- Levine, B. (2008) *The Art of Lobbying: Building Trust and Selling Policy* (Washington: CQ Press)
- Libby, P. (2011) *The Lobbying Strategy Handbook: 10 Steps to Advancing Any Cause Effectively* (London: Sage Publications)

m

marginalization

SEE ALSO civil society; community; empowerment; power; powerlessness; social justice

Marginalization is a process by which an individual or a group of individuals are denied access to, or positions of, economic, religious and political *power* within a society (Marshall, 1998).

Marginalization is relevant to health because marginalized groups often exist on the fringes of a society from where they can become excluded from, for example, access to services, and this can lead to poorer health. The circumstances of their marginalization, including poverty, discrimination and racism can contribute to their low self-esteem and to exclusion from main stream health promotion programmes. Marginalization can prevent people from participating in health and education services, are psychologically damaging and can lead to illness and premature death.

In practical terms, marginalized groups are considered to be those that are most in need, not able to meet their own needs, have a limited access to resources, are powerless or exist largely outside dominant social power structures. Marginalized groups not only include the elderly, the mentally ill and people of a low socio-economic status but can also be based on gender, ethnicity, (dis)ability and sexual preference. Although marginal groups are often a small population size relative to other groups in society they can actually be a numerical majority, for example, black people living in South Africa during apartheid (Laverack, 2009).

In the context of marginalization, Simpson and Yinger (1965) provide an early but relevant interpretation that does not place a numerical value on minority but its emphasis is on the social position of the group:

> Minorities are subordinate segments of complex state societies, have special physical or cultural traits that are held in low

esteem by the dominant segments of the society, are self-conscious units bound together by special traits which their members share (Simpson and Yinger, 1965, p. 17)

This *definition* also refers to the psychological status of the minority and their status within social power structures: do they feel themselves to be members of a particular social group that is clearly distinguished by them from other such groups? The group regard themselves as objects of collective discrimination having been singled out from the majority of others in the society in which they live, or by those who hold positions of power, for unequal treatment.

Ideally, health promoters work with those in greatest need and strive to avoid the establishment of a dominant minority. This requires some judgment on the part of the practitioner so that people coming forward as representatives of a *community* are in fact supported by its members and also have their best interest at heart.

Indigenous communities are a marginalized group to whom Simpson and Yinger's interpretation of a 'feeling of belonging or not belonging' has particular relevance. An example of indigenous communities living as a marginalized group within society is the Aboriginal and Torres Strait islander people in Australia. Today, Aboriginal communities are often a collection of families, language groups or clans who can be in competition over limited resources and who may have been traditionally geographically isolated. The term 'community' was applied to the formation of the settlements or 'Aboriginal reserves' by bureaucratic intellectuals and those in authority because it provided a convenient label for the assimilation of a heterogeneous group of people (Scrimgeour, 1997). Inevitably, these 'artificial' communities led to conflict, family feuds and violence fuelled by the frustration of a lack of opportunities, low income and access to alcohol.

Migrants are another example of marginalized groups. Migration, either in terms of internal migration where no national boundaries are crossed or international migration where people move to another place across national boundaries, occurs for a number of reasons. For example, people may leave their home to look for better economic opportunities, because of oppressive political circumstances, to be with family, for education or because they are forced to move. Migration is not always intended to be permanent and many people may wish to return to their home country at some stage in the future. A significant factor in the evolution of how migration patterns have developed has been advancements in travel (MacPherson and Gushulak, 2004). Migrant communities can become socially and economically marginalized and Simpson and Yinger's (1965) interpretation of a 'feeling of belonging or not belonging', discussed earlier, has resonance for many migrants. Examples of migrants living as a marginalized group within society include ethnic minorities such as Chinese and Turkish groups, religious groups such as Jewish and Muslim and illegal or seasonal workers. When living in a new country, many migrants are faced with restricted legal rights, a poor understanding of the local language, culture and system, different spiritual beliefs and a low income. This can lead to feelings of marginalization and alienation and as a consequence they can be placed in a more vulnerable position of poor physical and mental health. This is a situation that is compounded by some migrants having a limited understanding of how to access health care services (Laverack, 2009).

KEY TEXTS
- LaVeist, T. (2005) *Minority Populations and Health: An Introduction to Health Disparities in the US* (San Francisco, CA: Jossey-Bass)
- Laverack, G. (2009) *Public Health: Power, Empowerment and Professional Practice*. 2nd edn (Basingstoke: Palgrave Macmillan), Chapter 6
- Skrentny, J. (2004) *The Minority Rights Revolution* (Boston, MA: Belkap Press of Harvard University Press)

media

SEE ALSO advocacy; information and communication technologies; information, education and communication

The media refers collectively to technologies that are intended to reach a large audience via mass communication including printed materials, radio, television and the internet (Laverack, 2013).

The media offers an efficient and effective channel to reach both a large number of people or to target specific population groups. The media also offers low-cost options for communication as well as rapidly developing innovative methods with which to reach people at a local, national and international level. *The mass media* is an attractive option to health promoters because it can be used to reach a large number of people quickly and cheaply. This broad-based approach can be used to influence public opinion, both positively and negatively, to lobby and to raise the awareness of people about a particular cause. The use of the mass media is not an indiscriminate way to cover a large, ill-defined audience as messaging can be used to target specific audiences in much the same way that it is used by commercial advertising to reach specific age cohorts, income and social groups. Individuals not only receive the information through a mass media channel but may also watch and listen with family and friends, making it a social experience that can lead to discussion and action. Information received from the mass media can be quickly passed on through social networks, promoting debate and mass mobilization. The decline in smoking in the United Kingdom has been attributed to the use of vigorous anti-smoking campaigns both by the government and by *advocacy* groups. However, smoking decline has differed between social classes and this may have been because the mass media campaigns were targeted at the higher, better educated and professional social classes. For the mass media to achieve real change, it must be followed up with face-to-face communication, with a discussion or debate about the key issues, for example, by using printed materials. The mass media approach must also be carried out over a prolonged period of time and may require a generous budget to cover sophisticated advertising campaigns. The use of the mass media works best when the messaging is framed in a simple way, with a simple solution. The reinforcement of the mass media campaign from sympathetic journalistic coverage and the support from professional bodies will also help to increase the chances of success (Hubley, Copeman and Woodall, 2013).

Health promotion is not usually associated with scaremongering people into changing their behaviour, but the use of mass media 'fear appeals' is sometimes implemented, for example, to reduce smoking levels; otherwise, there is a threat of harmful consequences. A fear appeal involves threating the target audience with harmful outcomes for starting or continuing a particular high-risk behaviour such as drink-driving. Fear appeals can be an effective strategy when they are combined with an easy solution to rectify the harmful high-risk behaviour and this includes the inclusion of a problem-solving framework. However, mass media health promotion campaigns rarely allow for the necessary skills development to solve individual problems and instead confuse or increase fear within the target population groups (Corcoran, 2007, p. 93).

Community radio and television is based on the concept that the airwaves belong to everyone and provide a forum for people around the world to participate in social change. Community radio and television is a system that provides production equipment, training and airtime on local channels so that the public can produce programming and broadcast to a wide audience. Community radio and television offers access to broadcasting platforms to encourage diversity, creativity and participation in the media other than the ratings driven, market-oriented and privatized mass media. Community radio and television has been used by health promoters to focus on local as well as international issues using programme content that may be considered controversial. The development of community radio and television has been facilitated by technological change, which has made media broadcasting and production easier, cheaper and more accessible. Community television, for example in the United States, was assisted on a national level by federal regulations that were mandated as a result of the growth of the cable television industry in the early 1970s (Hackett, 2007). By 1972, the Federal Communications Commission authorized the creation of channels on new cable systems that would be available for state and local government, educational and community public access purposes. Cable companies would be required to provide studio space and equipment that could be used by any member of the community to broadcast on these public access channels. Community radio and television provide a range of programming including talk shows, education and cultural shows and a variety of entertainment channels. However, it also offers the space for rebuttal and debate on issues of free speech, decency and politics that may not be available in the mainstream mass media. Print materials include posters, leaflets, booklets and flip charts but can be used as a part of one-to-one communication to assist the transfer of information and skills when working with both literate and non-literate people.

Health promoters have also taken advantage of the world-wide web and the internet to become better communicators and social networkers using, for example, facebook, twitter, YouTube, the SMS and mobile telephones. These media communication tools have helped to extend participation, monitoring and transparency, to decentralize networks and provide opportunities to target individuals about specific health issues.

KEY TEXTS

- Corcoran, N. (ed) (2013) *Communicating Health: Strategies for Health Promotion.* 2nd edn (London: Sage Publications)
- Hanson, R.E. (2010) *Mass Communication: Living in a Media World* (Washington: CQ Press)
- Hubley, J., Copeman, J. and Woodall, J. (2013) *Practical Health Promotion.* 2nd edn (Cambridge, UK: Polity Press)

mental health promotion

SEE ALSO **determinants of health; empowerment; health social movements; individualism and health; lifespan approach; marginalization**

Mental health promotion involves actions to create conditions that support and maintain healthy lifestyles including mental health (WHO, 2001).

The field of mental health promotion is continuing to evolve, as is the *definition* of the term. Its definition is sometimes similar to that of health promotion 'the process of enhancing the capacity of individuals and communities to take control over their lives and improve their mental health using strategies that foster supportive environments and individual resilience, while showing respect for culture, equity, *social justice*, interconnections, and personal dignity' (Joubert, Taylor and Williams, 1996). However, it is important to understand that cross-cultural assumptions about the experience of mental health can be problematic.

Mental health can be described as a state of wellbeing in which an individual realizes that their abilities can cope with the normal stresses of life, can work productively and is able to make a contribution to his or her *community*. Multiple social, psychological and biological factors determine the level of mental health of a person. Poor mental health is associated with rapid social change, stressful work conditions, gender discrimination, social exclusion, unhealthy lifestyle, risks of violence and physical ill-health and human rights violations. There are also specific personality factors that make people vulnerable to mental disorders as well as genetic factors and imbalances in chemicals in the brain (WHO, 2001).

There is growing international evidence that mental ill health and poverty interact in a negative cycle, one that increases the likelihood that those living with mental illness will drift into or remain in poverty. This cycle applies to people with mental health issues living in poverty in high-income countries and people in low- and middle-income countries. Two principal causal pathways for this pattern are given: social causation and social drift. According to the social causation hypothesis, conditions of poverty increase the risk of mental illness through heightened stress, social exclusion, decreased social capital, malnutrition and increased obstetric risks, violence and trauma. Conversely, in the social drift hypothesis, people with mental illness are at increased risk of drifting into or remaining in poverty through increased health expenditure, reduced productivity, stigma and loss of employment and associated earnings. For example, the link between income and ill health is stronger for mental health than for general health. The social causation pathway might apply more readily to common mental disorders such as depression, whereas the social selection hypothesis might be more applicable to disorders such as schizophrenia and intellectual disabilities (Lund *et al.*, 2011).

Mental health promotion has a wide range of health, social and economic benefits including improved physical health, increased emotional resilience, greater social inclusion, higher employment and less poverty. A climate that respects and protects basic civil, political, socio-economic and cultural rights is fundamental to mental health promotion. Without the security and freedom provided by these rights, it is very difficult to maintain a high level of mental health. National mental health policies should not be solely concerned with mental disorders, but should also recognize and address the broader issues that promote mental health. This includes mainstreaming mental health promotion into policies and programmes in government and business sectors as well as the health sector (WHO, 2001).

Evidence exists for the effectiveness of a wide range of mental health promotion programmes and policies across the lifespan and across *settings* at the individual and community levels. Mental health programmes that target early childhood, for example, engage in interventions such as home visits for pregnant women, pre-school psycho-social activities and combined nutritional and psycho-social help for disadvantaged populations. The 'Prenatal and Infancy Home Visiting' programme, in the United States, impacted successfully on a range of behaviours including child abuse, conduct disorders and substance abuse. Parent training programmes such as 'The Incredible Years' and 'Triple P Positive Parenting' in Australia have improved parent–child interaction. Other programmes directly or indirectly address the mental health of communities such as 'Communities that Care' using multiple interventions to prevent violence and aggression (Sturgeon, 2007). Programmes that target unemployment and depression include the JOBS Programme, which has been tested and replicated in large-scale randomized trials in several countries. With regard to older people, controlled trials have demonstrated that exercise improves general mental wellbeing, and there is some evidence that befriending and early *screening* also have positive outcomes (Sturgeon, 2007). Other strategies for promoting mental health include those targeted at vulnerable groups, including minorities, indigenous people, migrants and people affected by conflicts and disasters (WHO, 2001).

Mental health groups have also unified themselves with a history of resistance against a dominant and unresponsive medical profession, which gives rise to feelings of an injustice as people living with mental illness struggle to gain more respect, dignity and autonomy (Allsop, Jones and Baggott, 2004). The collective action among mental health service users in Nottingham in England developed into a national advisory network and grew out of the meetings held by patients on hospital wards. While involved in the personal development of its members, the main aim of the group was to have an influence on shaping mental health policy and services (Barnes, 2002). Mad Pride is a mass movement and international network of mental health services, users and their allies who identify themselves as being psychiatric survivors, consumers and ex-patients. The movement started in response to local community prejudices towards people with a psychiatric history living in boarding homes in the Parkdale area of Toronto,

Canada. In the 1990s, similar protests and demonstrations were also being organized as Mad Pride events in England, Australia, South Africa and the United States. Mad Pride activists seek to reclaim terms such as 'mad', 'nutter' and 'psycho' from misuse by, for example, the *media*. Mad Pride has been successful in providing an opportunity to empower psychiatric survivors and raise public consciousness about human rights through various actions such as art, street theatre, music, poetry, protests and vigils (Mad Pride, 2013).

KEY TEXTS
- Cattan, M. and Tilford, S. (2006) *Mental Health Promotion. A Lifespan Approach* (Maidenhead: Open University Press)
- Sharma, M., Atri, A. and Branscum, P. (2011) *Foundations of Mental Health Promotion* (Boston, MA: Jones and Bartlett Learning)
- World Health Organization (2001) *Strengthening Mental Health Promotion* (Geneva: World Health Organization) Fact Sheet 220

moral suasion

SEE ALSO **alliances, partnerships and coalitions; behaviour change communication; leverage**

Moral suasion is the act of trying to use moral principles to influence individuals and groups to change their practices, beliefs and actions (Laverack, 2013, p. 148).

Persuasion is a process aimed at changing a person's (or a group's) attitude, belief or behaviour towards some other event or idea by using methods of communication including spoken words to convey information, feelings or reasoning. Persuasion can also be interpreted as using one's personal or positional resources to gain *leverage* to change people's behaviours or attitudes (Seiter and Gass, 2010). Moral suasion is a form of persuasion based on moral reasoning to change people's beliefs and behaviours. The temperance movement, for example, used a strategy of moral suasion to oppose the drinking of spirits and beer to the point of total abstinence in the United Kingdom in the nineteenth century. The strategy concentrated on the establishment of a mass movement of mostly working men to take a 'pledge' to cease from the use of alcohol. The movement offered support through a set of *self-help groups* and worked across the classes in society advocating for a sober workforce as well as for 'teetotallers' everywhere (Berridge, 2007).

A similar approach is with regard to foot-binding, universally practiced in China, it was painful and dangerous and afflicted Chinese women for a millennium. Yet this practice ended, for the most part, in a single generation. The natural-foot movement was championed by liberal modernizers and women's rights advocates and developed in the years of change culminating in the Revolution of 1911. Reform and urban economic development were part of modernization and mass migration from the countryside. This consequently provided alternative opportunities of support for women strengthening their independence and bargaining *power*. The natural-foot movement used moral suasion by forming alliances, called 'pledge associations', of parents who promised not to foot-bind their daughters nor let their sons marry foot-bound women (Mackie, 1996) as moral principles for the basis of individual behaviour change.

An important element in the process of mobilizing communities in the fight against female genital mutilation is moral suasion and the issue of a public statement or declarations as a decision to abandon Female Genital Mutilation (FGM) by a larger group, usually a significant part of a *community*. Public statements can take different forms, including signing a statement, alternative rites of passage celebrations and multi-village gatherings. When public statements are made, this suggests that a sufficient number of individuals have decided, on moral grounds, not to have their children cut and to abandon FGM, which can further promote broad-scale abandonment. The public statements, they can mark a final decision to abandon FGM or are a milestone that signifies readiness for change, and indicates that further support is needed to sustain and accelerate the process (Johansen *et al.*, 2013).

The limitation of persuasion techniques and moral suasion as an approach to health promotion is that it focuses on targeting individual behaviour change rather than broader structural change or through government intervention.

KEY TEXTS
- Berridge, V. (2007) 'Public Health Activism', *British Medical Journal*, 335: pp. 1310–1312

- Johansen, E. *et al.* (2013) 'What Works and What Does Not: A Discussion of Popular Approaches for the Abandonment of Female Genital Mutiliation', *Obstetrics and Gynaecology International*. Advance access ID 348248
- Mackie, G. (1996) 'Ending Footbinding and Infibulation: A Convention Account', *American Sociological Review*, 61 (6): pp. 999–1017

n

needs assessment

SEE ALSO community-based interventions; health profiles; lay epidemiology; photo-voice

Needs assessment can be defined as a process that is used to identify the needs reported by an individual or group (Gilmore, 2011). More specifically, a health needs assessment is a systematic procedure for determining the unmet health and health care needs of a population, the causes and contributing factors to those needs and the human, organizational and *community* resources, which are available to respond to these needs (Wright, 2001).

Needs assessment is a logical starting point in the design of a health promotion programme. It essentially identifies what society values, and what resources and outcomes are required to meet their needs as a part of the programme design. A needs assessment approach involves an epidemiological and qualitative approach for determining priorities and determines what should be done, what can be done and what can be afforded. The stages in the needs assessment approach include mapping, the identification, ranking and prioritization of the causes of problems and the solutions to resolve them. Too rigid an approach runs the real risk of becoming top-down and controlling, while too flexible an approach runs the risk of delay or not having a direction in which to move forward. Felt and expressed health needs assessment is useful for the planning of health promotion programmes and for the active involvement of all stakeholders, including community members, in decisions about how needs should be effectively addressed (Jirojwong and Liamputtong, 2009).

There are a number of strategies that can be used for needs assessment in health promotion work, for example, mapping is a visual means of providing information with regard to a community need. The visual aspect helps people to understand the issues at all levels and to find ways in which to solve them. Maps are commonly geographical, concerning the physical layout of a community, or social, identifying the people and where they are situated. Mapping can be done in a collective or on an individual basis (Rifkin and Pridmore, 2001). The purpose is to allow people to better understand, through a textual or a visual means, how they can build their resource base from an existing position of strength. The role of the practitioner is to act as a guide to encourage the community to think critically about what are their own strengths, their access to external resources and their ability to make decisions.

Once the needs have been identified, it is the role of the practitioner to help the community to rank them and then to move towards decision making and action. Ranking is a simple exercise to 'unpack' the many complex issues that influence people's lives into its different elements so that they can be ordered, further analysed and then addressed. When working with clients who are non-literate, pictures or drawings can be used instead of words to develop a ranked list. The prioritized list can then be scored, placing the highest at the top of the list and the lowest score to the need at the bottom of the list.

While there are many methodologies for assessing individual and community needs, the following is an innovative approach that has achieved some success. The grounded citizens' jury is an approach for local involvement in health needs assessment and decision making. For example, the concerns identified by people in South West Burnley, UK, using this approach included the following: low pay; poor housing and an increasing number of empty and derelict properties; increasing alcohol abuse by children; high crime levels, especially drug-related burglaries; poor access to health and social services; teenage pregnancies and a high volume of fast moving traffic and accidents (Kashefi and Mort, 2004).

The process begins when a steering committee selects 12–16 citizens to form the jury. These jury members are selected because they can offer an opinion on the health needs of their community and not because they represent a particular section or organization. For example, jury members may be single mothers, the elderly, unemployed or people from an average family with children. The jury meets for a 4–5 day period, with the purpose of reaching a 'verdict' on a particular long-standing problem regarding local circumstances and service provision related to the health needs of its citizens. The jury is posed a general question such as 'what would improve the *health and wellbeing* of residents in your community.' The jury undergoes a period of training in preparation for the meeting and are given time to asks questions about their roles and responsibilities. To help the jury it hears the testimonies from local health and welfare workers, members are presented with the results of data collected about community opinions such as focus groups with school children and may meet with local community groups before further deliberation and the preparation of a report. The commissioning agency is committed to respond and take action on some of the recommendations made by the jury. The jury members are not practitioners or researchers and their deliberations can result in many recommendations that cover pertinent local concerns. Prioritization is therefore an important step in focusing the jury onto a few key needs and the solutions that they are able to recommend such as improved service provision. Follow-up to the jury recommendations by the steering committee and the inclusion of jury members in this process of further development is a key point for the success of the approach.

Other strategies for needs assessment include using existing data (quantitative and qualitative), survey and questionnaire methods, observation techniques, in-depth interviewing, rapid rural appraisal, *photo-voice* and participatory community-based techniques. However, it should be noted that a limitation of using techniques for needs assessment as the starting point for informed community choices is that they require skilled facilitation and a long-term commitment. Within a health promotion programme, this may not always be realistic to achieve because of financial and time constraints and because of a lack of professional competence and confidence in using these types of *approaches*.

KEY TEXTS
- Gilmore, G. (2011) *Needs and Capacity Assessment for Health Education and Health Promotion.* 4th edn (Boston, MA: Jones and Bartlett Learning)
- Jirojwong, S. and Liamputtong, P. (eds) (2009) *Population Health, Communities and Health Promotion* (Oxford: Oxford University Press), Chapter 3

- Rifkin, S.B. and Pridmore, P. (2001) *Partners in Planning: Information, Participation and Empowerment* (London: MacMillan Education)

networks

SEE ALSO **alliances, partnerships and coalitions; health social movements; patient empowerment**

Networks set a context within groups, formal organizations and institutions for those who work in or are served by them, which, in turn, affects what people do, how they feel and what happens to them (Wright, 1997).

A network is a structure of relationships linking social actors (Wasserman and Faust, 1994) that in turn are the building blocks of human experience, mapping the connections that individuals have to one another (Pescosolido, 1991). Social structures are not based therefore on categorizations such as age, gender or race but on the actual nature of the social contacts that individuals have and the impact on people's lives (White, 1992). A health network is a structure of relationships, both personal and professional, through which individuals maintain and receive emotional support, resources, services and information for the improvement of their *health and wellbeing* (Walker *et al.*, 1977). These networks can be an indication of related health behaviour, for example, the biological and behavioural traits associated with obesity appear to be spread through social ties. People who experience the weight gain of others in their social networks may then more readily accept weight gain in themselves. Moreover, social distance was more important than geographic distance within networks and there was an important role for a process involving the induction and person-to-person spread of obesity. Peer support interventions that allow for a modification of people's social networks are therefore more successful than those that do not. Social networks can also be used to spread positive health behaviours because people's perceptions of their own risk of illness may depend on the people around them (Christakis and Fowler, 2007).

In a fundamental way, our health is a reflection of the quality of our relationships with one another and social networks offer many people the opportunity to strengthen the level of social capital in their lives. *Social capital* in the form of trust, social norms of reciprocity and cooperation resides in relationships, not individuals, and therefore in the social networks in which they participate. Active participation within social networks builds the trust and cohesiveness between individuals that are important to mobilize and create the resources necessary to support collective action. Social capital is a feature of social organization such as networks, trust, facilitated co-ordination and collaboration. Individuals invest in and use the resources embedded in social networks because they expect returns of some sort, although resources are not equally available to all individuals and are differentially distributed across groups in society (Lin, 2000).

The Patients Association (UK), for example, is a network about common patient issues for better information and support. The most frequent complaints received by the Patients Association are poor communication; toileting; pain relief; nutrition and hydration. The Association addresses the shared concerns of its members including the 'duty to refer', for patients to be able to trust that their doctors are making sure they are getting access to the best treatment. Access to information is the best way to make sure this is happening and patient support groups are ideally placed to provide this service. Doctors cannot be experts in all fields and so it is important for them to be able to direct patients to other organizations that have the expertise. Doctors can then actively support patients in finding support groups and networks that could help them with managing their condition (Patients Association, 2011).

Networks also have some features that are particularly relevant to professional groups such as health promotion, whose functions rely on the interactions between its members. Social relationships underpin network activity with a strong sense of professional identity and solidarity and offer individuals and organizations the opportunity to access complementary resources and expertise. However, networks require significant investment for their establishment and maintenance and may therefore absorb rather than unlock resources, at least in the short term. Networks require a non-hierarchical management style that allows an interaction between its members, and this is in contrast to the bureaucratic and hierarchical style of much of the health promotion sector.

KEY TEXTS

- Christakis, N.A. and Fowler, J.H. (2007) 'The Spread of Obesity in a Large Social Network over 32 Years', *New England Journal of Medicine,* 357 (4): pp. 370–379
- Pescosolido, B.A. (1991) 'Illness Careers and Network Ties: A Conceptual Approach of Utilization and Compliance' in G. Albrecht and J. Levy (eds), *Advances in Medical Sociology* (Greenwich, CT: JAI Press), pp. 161–184
- Wasserman, S. and Faust. K.B. (1994) *Social Network Analysis: Methods and Applications* (New York: Cambridge University Press)

p

parallel-tracking

SEE ALSO approaches; bottom-up and top-down; community capacity building; empowerment; photo-voice

Parallel-tracking is a planning framework that uses a multi-stage approach to view the top-down and bottom-up tensions in health promotion programming in a uniquely different way (Laverack, 2007, p. 47).

The parallel-tracking framework moves our thinking on from a simple bottom-up/top-down dichotomy, and helps to formalize bottom-up objectives and processes within more conventional top-down health promotion programmes (Laverack, 2004). The processes of capacity building and *empowerment* are viewed as a 'parallel track' running alongside the main 'programme track'. The tensions between the two, rather than being conventionally viewed as a top-down versus a bottom-up situation, can now occur at each stage of the programme cycle, making their resolution much easier. The framework is normally initiated by health promoters who are genuinely concerned with empowerment and programme sustainability. Their incentive is to utilize *approaches* to build capacities that can lead both to the continued management of programmes and to increased *community* abilities to 'take greater control over' the important health determinants in their lives, even if these are not initially part of programme objectives.

The issue at stake is how the programme and the empowerment tracks become linked during the progressive stages of the programme cycle. The framework poses questions to assist health promoters to identify the tensions that can exist between the two tracks when accommodating empowerment into each stage of the programme cycle: (1) overall programme design; (2) objective setting; (3) strategy selection; (4) strategy implementation and management and (5) programme *evaluation*.

Overall programme design

The first opportunity where the 'top-down' and 'bottom-up' tensions can begin to resolve is in the design characteristics of the programme itself. Specifically, programme design, regardless of its content, can be made more empowering by using strategic and participatory planning approaches. Such approaches allow the involvement of the participants and help to resolve conflicts that may arise later during implementation and *evaluation*. In this context, the concept of the programme itself changes. Rather than being a time-limited or 'one-off' educational or marketing activity, the programme becomes essentially a vehicle through which longer term relationships between the health promotion agency and community members are built. Through this relationship, various financial, material, human and knowledge resources become available to community members and help to enhance their capacity to act on specific short-term issues.

Objective setting

In conventional health promotion programming, objectives are developed during the design phase and are usually centred on *disease prevention*, a reduction in morbidity and mortality and lifestyle management such as a change in specific health-related behaviours. The issue is how to give empowerment objectives equal priority with disease prevention programmes. Empowerment objectives are usually centred on a gain in control over decisions influencing choices, for example, over the *determinants of health* and are likely to change as peoples experiences of capacity and *power* increase over time. This 'learning-in-action' is what typifies the more 'bottom-up' or empowering approaches to health promotion. Broad health concerns that might be expressed initially by groups, for example, reducing poverty in a given locality, may change as the group engages in activities towards this long-term goal. Through strategies such as dialogue and problem analysis, the group may decide to narrow its focus towards more immediate and resolvable issues, for example, improving living conditions in public housing.

Strategy selection

It is important that the strategy used by the programme should also strengthen the empowerment objectives to improve the quality of social relations, capacity and positive perceptions. For example, theories on change in community through collective action (diffusion of innovation theory, community organization and capacity building) provide opportunities for *community-based intervention*, empowerment and addressing the broader socio-economic determinants of health. The socio-environmental approach to health promotion focuses on how people can move to influence high-risk social and environmental conditions including the structural causes of health inequality.

Strategy implementation and management

Health promoters require both the practical methodologies and examples of 'good practice' for the assessment and strategic planning of community empowerment in a programme context. Community participation is very important to ensure that strategy implementation and management is also an empowering practice. The management of health promotion programmes should ideally be steered by the expressed needs and involvement of the community, facilitated by the sympathetic role of the health promoter, to allow the community, at least in part, to develop its own actions and activities. This can have a strong positive effect on the confidence of the community members who will also feel that this, in turn, has had a positive influence on their health (Smithies and Webster, 1998).

Programme evaluation

Community empowerment can be a long and slow process. Particular outcomes in the community empowerment process may not occur until many years after the programme time frame has been completed. Thus, the evaluation of community empowerment within a programme context, which has a limited time frame, can more appropriately assess changes in the process rather than any particular outcome. In effect, success in the process become the outcomes. The health promotion programme design can therefore be made more empowering when using participatory evaluation approaches that involve the experiences of the community.

KEY TEXTS

- Laverack, G. and Labonte, R. (2000) 'A Planning Framework for Accommodation of Community Empowerment Goals within Health

Promotion Programming', *Health, Policy and Planning*, 15 (3): pp. 255–262
- Laverack, G. (2004) *Health Promotion Practice: Power and Empowerment* (London: Sage Publications), Chapter 6

patient empowerment

SEE ALSO **advocacy; disease prevention; empowerment; individualism and health; networks; power**

Patient empowerment includes enabling individuals to take control of their own health, wellbeing and disease management and participate in decisions affecting their care. Patient empowerment is also about respecting patients' rights, giving them a 'voice' so that they can actively and collectively participate in making health systems more user friendly and information more accessible (The Lancet, 2012).

Patient empowerment is different to the traditional, paternalistic approach to care that tends to ignore personal preferences, and creates dependency because it does not focus on patient-centred care. Patient empowerment can therefore be in conflict with the ideology of the health practitioner–patient relationship. This professional relationship is traditionally paternalistic and unequal where all competence and expertise is considered to belong to the person with the control, the health practitioner. An example of the delicate balance at an individual level can be illustrated in the doctor–patient relationship. The doctor (after an examination) tells the patient what their medical problem is and prescribes a treatment for it. The patient voluntarily surrenders to the unspoken claim of medical (expert) power, for example, the phrase 'Doctor knows best' epitomizes this situation. The doctor has control over the knowledge, even though this concerns the patient's own body. The attributes of health are viewed as an individual 'case' and the diagnosis is made on the basis of the medical approach (the presence or absence of disease or illness) that serves to protect the legitimate and expert bases of power held by the doctor. However, in the health system, the power-over relationship does not stop at diagnosis because the doctor often also controls the admission and discharge, choice of treatment, referral and care of the patient (Laverack, 2007). A more equal relationship would be the one in which the doctor uses their knowledge to allow the patient to make informed decisions about their treatment and recovery. In effect, the patient is placed at the centre of the issue requiring the doctor to gain as much information as possible from their experience rather than what the doctor should achieve in the consultation.

The patient-centred clinical method applies the principles of *empowerment* in a practitioner–patient relationship as follows:

1. The illness and the patient's experience of being ill are explored at the same time.
2. Understanding the person as a whole places the illness into context by considering: How does the illness affect the person? How does the person interact with their immediate environment? How does the wider environment influence this interaction?
3. The patient and doctor reach a mutual understanding on the nature of the illness its causes and its goals for management, and who is responsible for what.
4. The desirability and applicability to undertake broader health promoting and illness prevention tasks, for example, providing the patient with information or skills about how he/she themselves can dress a wound at home.
5. Gaining a better understanding of the patient–doctor relationship in order to enhance it, for example, placing a value on the contribution being made by both sides and forming a 'partnership' to address the illness rather than a traditional paternalistic approach.
6. Making a realistic assessment of what can be done to help the patient given, for example, constraints in understanding, time and skill level (Stewart *et al.*, 2003).

Chronic disease management is not intended to substitute professional acute care, but by learning to self-manage, people with chronic diseases are more likely to remain integrated into society and the workforce. Chronic disease self-management can support individuals to gain confidence and acquire the skills to recognize warning symptoms, take medication and decide the treatment that is best suited to them (The Lancet, 2012). Giving the patient more control over their recovery can also occur as part of home-based treatment and care for the dying. One study (Bassett and Prapavessis, 2007) on physical therapy for ankle sprains showed that the home-based groups had similar outcome scores for post-treatment ankle function, adherence and motivation to a standard physical therapy intervention. However, the home-based group had significantly better attendance at clinic appointments and a better physical therapy completion rate. Patients were helped to set goals and to develop personal action plans to complete the therapy as well as education and skills training on the treatment such as strapping techniques. The patients had more control and were better informed about their recovery and this sharing of knowledge and skills led to a viable home-based option. Nevertheless, self-care can be a complicated issue that is not appropriate for all situations or people and the importance of arranging for patients to choose the nature or timing of treatment, or teaching them 'coping skills' in groups has shown variable results (Salmon and Hall, 2004).

Patient empowerment interventions are unlikely to be successful unless health practitioners understand a fundamental principle: before they can empower others, they must first be themselves empowered and understand the sources of their own *power*. To build a more empowering practice, the constraints placed on the profession by its institutional nature and culture that do not share an ideology of empowerment must be redressed. This has been argued in the context of a nursing profession that cannot be empowered unless individual nurses themselves are empowered and can be extended to an institutional work setting such as a hospital: a *community* of both patients and staff. Both must be empowered and this includes feeling valued and having the resources, skills and knowledge to empower others (Kendall, 1998). Nurses work to enable patients to take more control in decision making over their health, promoting patient independence, information exchange and being aware of their needs. In practice, this translates into acts of care such as making sure patients had their call bell within reach, respecting their choices, providing information about future care options and working quietly at night to allow patients to sleep (Faulkner, 2001). This is an individualistic approach that gives credibility to what the individual has to offer self-care.

The broader empowerment of patients enable them to also have an influence on the health system through networking and engagement with *advocacy* and *pressure groups*. Patient Advocacy Groups, for example, allow people to represent others and to speak out for their rights as patients. One Patient Advocacy Group in a UK hospital was established to allow comments and concerns to be raised anonymously and to have feedback about actions taken. Patients and their carers were given comment forms, which could be returned to a member of staff or placed in a collection box. Once a month, all of the comments, both positive and negative, were reviewed by the advocacy group and action was decided upon at an appropriate level, or a report given about action already taken. The results of each action were posted on display boards in the wards to inform the patients and their carers and of the actions taken. These included side rooms for infection control had curtains fitted with curtains to act as a screen, wards that suffered from solar glare received vertical blinds to improve conditions and shelves were put up in bathrooms to help patients to manage their own care. Each ward was asked to nominate representatives of whom one would be available to attend each monthly meeting. The number of formal complaints decreased to less than 20% of the previous level as patients gained confidence that their comments would be acted upon and that the ward environment had improved (Improvement Network, 2011). Patient *networks* can be formed by its members for the benefit of its members, both patients and health practitioners, and can be the means through which people can become empowered through better communication and organization. Patient Concern (UK), for example, operates a network in collaboration with other active groups run by patients and volunteers on issues that matter to them, including protection for whistleblowers, assisted suicide, campaigns against the reduction of hospital beds and strengthening complaints procedures (Patient Concern, 2012).

Patient empowerment should involve both collective action and individual self-care, to enable people to have more of a 'voice' about the health care that they receive and, more importantly, to be able to take action if this does not meet their needs and expectations.

KEY TEXTS

- Frampton, S., Charmel, P. and Plantree, C. (eds) (2008) *Putting Patients First: Best Practice in Patient Centered Care* (San Francisco, CA: Jossey-Bass)
- Godbold, N. and Vaccarella, M. (2012) *Autonomous, Responsible, Alone: The Complexities of Patient empowerment* (Freeland, Oxfordshire: Interdisciplinary Press)
- Stewart, M.A. *et al.* (2003) *Patient Centred Medicine: Transforming the Clinical Method.* 2nd edn (Oxford: Radcliffe Medical Publications)

peer education

SEE ALSO **behaviour change communication; counselling and one-to-one communication; information, education and communication**

Peer education is an approach in which people are supported to promote health-enhancing change among their peers. Rather than health professionals educating members of the public, lay persons are felt to be in the best position to encourage healthy behaviour to each other (Kelly *et al.*, 1992).

In health promotion, peer education is usually initiated by practitioners who recruit members of the 'target' *community* to serve as educators. Peer educators are typically about the same age as the group with whom they are working. The recruited peer educators are trained in relevant health information and communication skills and then engage their peers in conversations about the issue of concern, seeking to promote health-enhancing behaviour change. The intention is that familiar people, giving locally relevant and meaningful suggestions, in a local language and taking account of the local context, will be more likely to promote health. They may work alongside the health promoter, run educational activities on their own or actually take the lead in organizing and implementing activities. Youth peer educators, for example, have shown in some cases to be more effective than adults in establishing norms and in changing attitudes related to sexual behaviour (UNICEF, 2013).

Peer education has become very popular in the field of HIV prevention, especially involving young people, sex workers, men who have sex with men and intravenous drug users. Peer education is also associated with efforts to prevent tobacco, drug or alcohol use among young people, teenage pregnancy and home-lessness. The Alcohol and Substance Abuse Prevention (ASAP) programme, for example, sought to empower youth from high-risk populations to make healthier choices in their own lives and to play active political and social roles in society. The programme approach brought small groups of high-school students together in a hospital emergency centre and a county detention centre to interact with patients and detainees who had drug-related problems. Youth were able to share experiences directly with the inmates and with their peers to learn through asking ques-tions and exploring problems at different levels. The students formed a 'Students Against Drunk Driving (SADD)' chapter when one of the students was killed in a drink-related driving accident. Gradually the students began to take a *leadership* role and organized meetings and events to raise the issues of drug abuse and drink driving in local meetings. The students had a statistically significant increase in self-reported perception of the risks involving drinking and drug abuse as compared to the control group, which showed a significant drop in perception (Wallerstein and Bernstein, 1988).

Despite its popularity, the evidence about peer education is mixed, seemingly working in some contexts but not in others. One study comparing peer education among sex workers in India and South Africa, for example, found that the more successful Indian group benefited from a supportive social and political context, and a more effective community development ethos, rather than the biomedical focus of the South African intervention (Cornish and Campbell, 2009).

Peer education should be seen as a strategy that can be used alongside other strategies in a broader health promotion approach or community-wide effort. For example, it has been used effectively to complement skills-based *health education* on condom promotion and youth-friendly health services (UNICEF, 2013).

KEY TEXTS
- Robertson, J., Catanzarite, J. and Hong, L. (2010) *Peer Health Education: Concepts and Content* (San Diego, CA: University Readers)
- UNICEF (2013) Peer education, http://www.unicef.org/lifeskills/ index_12078.html [accessed 21/1/2013]

photo-voice

SEE ALSO **critical consciousness; empowerment; political activity; power**

Photo-voice is a tool to enable people to identify, represent and enhance their *community* through a specific photographic technique. It entrusts cameras to people to enable them to act as recorders and potential catalysts for social action and change, in their own communities (Photo-voice, 2013).

Photo-voice can be used to reach, inform and organize community members, enabling them to prioritize their concerns and discuss problems and solutions. Photo-voice uses the immediacy of the visual image and accompanying stories to furnish evidence and to promote an effective, participatory means of sharing experiences and local knowledge to resolve problems. It goes beyond the conventional role of community assessment by inviting people to promote their own and their community's well-being. It is a 'tool' that enables people to define for themselves and others, including policy makers, what is worth remembering and what needs to be changed.

Photo-voice has two main goals:

1. To enable people to record and reflect their community's strengths and concerns;
2. To promote critical dialogue and knowledge about personal and community issues through group discussions of photographs (Photo-voice, 2013).

People using photo-voice engage in a three-stage process that provides the foundation for analyzing the pictures they have taken:

Stage 1. Selecting: Choosing those photographs that most accurately reflect the community's concerns and assets. So that people can lead the discussion, it is they who choose the photographs. They select photographs they consider most significant, or simply like best, from each picture they had taken.

Stage 2. Contextualizing or story telling: The participatory approach also generates the second stage, contextualizing or storytelling. This occurs in the process of group discussion, voicing our individual and collective experience. Photographs alone, considered outside the context of their own voices and stories, would not add to the essence of photo-voice. People therefore have to describe the meaning of their images in group discussions and it is this that provides meaning and context.

Stage 3. Codifying: The participatory approach gives multiple meanings to singular images and thus frames the third stage, codifying. In this stage, participants may identify three types of dimensions that arise from the dialogue process: issues, themes or theories. The individual or group may codify issues when the concerns targeted for action are pragmatic, immediate and tangible. This is the most direct application of the analysis. The individual or group may also codify themes or develop theories that are grounded in a more systematic analysis of the images.

Photo-voice has been used to promote community action in, for example, St. Jamestown, an established immigrant-receiving area of great ethno-racial diversity in Toronto. It is the most densely populated area in Canada with 64,000 people living in old high-rise rental apartment buildings. The photo-voice approach was used to help newcomer communities influence public policy, secure improved local services and enhance existing community strengths that promote *health and wellbeing*. Images of community issues were taken using a camera by people living in the area and then an account was created to explain what was important in the picture using their own words. The resident action group displayed the images at a 'Community Forum and Exposition', attended by over 300 people. It was decided by the action group to then take these issues to the City Counsellor's office. The recommendations made to the city authorities were modest and related to day-to-day living issues affecting all age groups in the neighbourhood. Bicycle theft due to improperly maintained bicycle racks was identified as a common problem. Since biking is the main mode of transport for many residents in this neighbourhood, safe bicycle storage is a daily stressor for many people. The action group worked with the city authorities to take an inventory of all bicycle racks, arrange the removal of broken bicycles from existing racks and install new racks in the neighbourhood. The decision of city authorities to remove broken and abandoned bicycles from the neighbourhood was as of a direct result of the photo-voice approach. The group was successful in advocating for changes that required intervention at the city level but the broader issues such as employment opportunities, recognition of foreign qualifications, housing repairs and health care accessibility remained unaddressed (Haque and Eng, 2011).

Having an influence on the broader causes of poverty and *powerlessness*, for example, unemployment and social exclusion, has not been achieved using photo-voice because these require further political commitment. Photo-voice is a 'tool' that can help to engage community members in *needs assessment*, asset mapping and programme planning and to assist people to advocate for social and political change.

KEY TEXTS
- Photo-voice (2013) 'Social Change through Photography', www. photo-voice.org. [accessed 5/3/2013]
- Wang, C. *et al.* (1998) 'Photo-Voice as a Participatory Health Promotion Strategy', *Health Promotion International*, 13 (1): pp. 75–86

political activity

SEE ALSO **empowerment; global health; healthy public policy; individualism and health; leverage; lobbying; power**

Health promotion is, or should be, a political activity, as many of its actions have political consequences for those in the society in which it occurs. Health promotion actions, for example, attempt to influence people at an individual, civic and political level with regard to the development of health-related legislation and policy. Health promotion aims at enabling others to take more control of their lives, health and its determinants through social, economic and political change. To be more politically effective, practitioners must fully understand the sources of their own *power* and how this can be used to help to empower others (Laverack, 2004). Political ideology too influences who is responsible for health (the individual or the state) and as a consequence who is responsible for regulating behaviour and behaviour change (Dixey *et al.*, 2013).

Those in politics, those who govern and who have decision making control, can be supportive (democratic, liberal and egalitarian) towards health promotion and provide channels for the meaningful participation of *civil society*. In these circumstances, there is a clear and constitutional separation of political parties, the legal system, corporate and church authorities (Baum, 2008). The social democratic model, for example, has been most committed to economic and social policies and supportive of public health and *community* action in developed countries (Navarro and Shi, 2001). Other circumstances are even more likely to address social injustice and health inequality and include the following:

- the presence of 'left' political parties to influence government decision making;
- proportional representation electoral systems that increase the likelihood of such a presence;
- an historic state commitment to active labour policy, support for women's employment, adequate spending to support families, assistance for the unemployed and those with disabilities, provision of educational and recreational opportunities and efforts to reduce social exclusion and promote democratic participation;
- high union density and effective labour powers to negotiate favourable wage and employment conditions and
- the presence of strong civil society organizations with similar commitments (Bryant, 2006).

Unsupportive circumstances (undemocratic, authoritarian and inegalitarian) in contrast have closed *leadership*, are authoritarian and are highly regimented, often with just one political party and no free and fair electoral or legal system (Baum, 2008). Under these circumstances, people must seize control through collective action, first at a localized level, and then through broader social and political change, making strategic decisions about what tactics they can use. Oppressive forms of governance, dominated by elite group interests, does not allow civil society to function but neither can people rely upon support from the state to promote their *health and wellbeing*. Community action is tightly controlled and people must therefore use the only significant resource they have, the capacity to cause trouble. The tactics used are unconventional and increasingly disruptive, but the civil disobedience, public support and the reaction of the government become the basis for political influence.

It is a risky option but one that historically has given rise to significant social and political change, for example, the 'Arab Spring' in North Africa (Abulof, 2011).

People can conventionally express their discontent with the political situation by attending a local planning meeting, voting, signing a petition or writing a letter to lobby someone in a decision-making position. However, those who are low on the social gradient are often unsuccessful in using these indirect strategies because they lack the resources and political *leverage* necessary to have an influence. People who can persuade others to make changes do so by using direct tactics that include a show of support, for example, through mass demonstrations. These actions are partly symbolic, challenging government decisions and sending a message to politicians and policymakers about their grievances. The purpose is to shift political opinion about a particular decision, especially when it favours one group's interests or has not yet arrived at a firm view on an issue.

Global economic conditions, for example, at the beginning of the twenty-first century, have given rise to many governments pursuing an even tighter neo-liberal agenda. Public policies have been promoted that reduce social and economic structures, deregulate labour and financial markets and stimulate commerce and investment (Navarro, 2009). For everyday living conditions, this means that governments are cutting pay and jobs, freezing benefits and welfare payments and reducing opportunities for *empowerment*, education and maintenance of the infrastructure (Nathanson and Hopper, 2010). Governments are further reducing their responsibility by increasing market choice, transforming national health services into insurance-based health care systems, privatizing medical care and promoting a bio-medical model of health towards individual behaviour change (Navarro, 2009).

Empowerment is central to health promotion practice and involves people gaining control to influence economic, political and social change, in their favour. For example, by changing health and welfare policy to support those who are on a low income, are unemployed or who have a disability. 'Every Australian Counts' is a civil society campaign for a National Disability Insurance Scheme in Australia. The scheme will be a new support system for people with a disability, their families and carers to ensure people are better supported and to enable them to have greater choice and control. The campaign purposefully coincided with the Productivity Commission report to the Australian Government on the findings of its inquiry into a long-term disability care and support scheme. The campaign is designed to lobby government and to advocate for change in the existing system using information sharing, supporter registration forms and links to facebook and twitter. *Lobbying* targets politicians and other influential people and recruits 'champions' to support their cause such as *media* personalities (Every Australian Counts, 2012).

Resistance by civil society is especially important when governments are pursuing a tighter political and economic agenda to involve people in a struggle with those already holding power. Health promotion practitioners must recognize that an empowering approach to their work is also a political activity. To Rudolf Virchow, for example, there was no distinction between being a health professional and a political activist, 'All disease has two causes,' he once wrote, 'one pathological and the other political' (Laverack, 2004, p. 2). The political nature of health promotion is extended even further when faced with the challenges of the global transfer of health risks as a result of an expansion of the movement of people, environmental threats, lifestyle changes and the trade in harmful products (Parker and Sommer, 2011).

The structures of power-over, bureaucracy and authority remain dominant and the role of the practitioner, at least in part, is to strive to help others to challenge these circumstances. This role is explicitly driven by goals for political change manifest as new or favourable changes to policy and legislation. Practitioners have the right and therefore an option of exercising their own voices as citizens, for example, through their participation in social movements. In the same way, practitioners can act as professional advocate groups to support the actions of others who they believe suffer from a health inequality. They can endorse the concerns of these less powerful groups by using their 'expert power' to legitimize their concerns. For example, the support of the medical profession to the *advocacy* group 'Action on Smoking and Health' has given credibility to its cause and in some European countries has contributed to a nationwide ban on passive smoking in public places. Likewise, the British Medical Association has given its support to the political lobby for the stricter legal regulation of boxing (Brayne *et al.*, 1998) based on health grounds.

KEY TEXTS

- Baum, F. (2008) *The New Public Health.* 3rd edn (Australia and New Zealand: Oxford Higher Education)
- Dixey, R. *et al.* (2013) *Health Promotion: Global Principles and Practice* (Wallingford, Oxfordshire: CAB International)
- Naidoo, J. and Wills, J. (2009) *Foundations for Health Promotion.* 3rd edn (Edinburgh: Bailliere and Tindall), Chapter 7

population health

SEE **public health**

power

SEE ALSO **empowerment; health activism; health social movements; hegemonic power; moral suasion; political activity; powerlessness**

The common interpretation of power is simply as '...the capacity of some to produce intended and foreseen effects on others' (Wrong, 1988, p. 2).

The aforementioned interpretation is a common variation of how power is referenced in the social science literature: One person having influence and mastery over another. To exercise choice is the simplest form of power. This may involve the trivial choices of everyday life or the more critical choices that influence health. To the extent our personal choices constrain those of others, it becomes an exercise of power-over. For example, people with the ability to control decisions at the political and economic level condition and constrain the ability of other people to exercise choice at the individual and group levels. Sometimes we willingly accord people this 'higher' level ability, such as legislation to prevent or punish people, to protect the health of others (Laverack, 2004).

In contrast to hard power, 'soft power' is the ability to obtain what one wants through indirect and long-term actions such as co-option and attraction. The purpose is to persuade others to voluntarily do what you want them to do avoiding conflict and tension. The primary currencies of soft power are values, culture, policies and institutions, agenda control and the extent to which these are able to attract or repel others. The phrase 'you are either with us or against us' is an exercise in soft power, since no explicit threat is included. However, rationalists would argue that this is an 'implied threat' and that direct economic or military sanctions would likely follow. The success of soft power can depend on one person's reputation as well as on the flow of information. *Media* is regularly identified as a source of soft power, as is the spread of a national language, or a particular set of normative values (Gallarotti, 2011, p. 27). An example of soft power is *moral suasion*, the use of moral principles to influence individuals and groups to change their practices, beliefs and actions (Berridge, 2007). Because soft power has appeared as an alternative to hard power, it is often not only embraced by ethically minded scholars and policymakers, but has also been criticized as being ineffective and too difficult to distinguish between the effects of other factors. The difference between soft and hard power is that the latter achieves compliance through direct and coercive methods and by compelling others to do what you want them to do, whether they want to do it or not.

To better understand how power is exercised in both a positive (the sharing of control with others) and a negative manner (the use of control to exert influence over others against their will), it is helpful to consider three of its simplest forms: 'power-from-within'; 'power-over' and 'power with'.

Power-from-within can be described as an experience of 'self', a personal or psychological power. The many definitions of this concept, developed in the field of psychology in westernized countries, describe it as gaining (a sense of) control over one's life (Rissel, 1994). Starhawk's (1990, p. 10) description of power-from-within is similar; she likens it to '... our sense of mastery we develop as young children ...', but also to something deeper '... our sense of bonding with other human beings, and with the environment'. The goal is to increase feelings of value and a sense of individual mastery and to increase the notion of 'self', without access to or control over resources. Individuals can therefore become more powerful from within and do not necessarily have to accumulate power as money, status or authority.

Power-over describes social relationships in which one party is made to do what another party wishes them to, despite their resistance and even if it may not be in their best interests. Starhawk

(1990, p. 9) describes power-over in its most direct form as '...the power of the prison guard, of the gun, power that is ultimately backed by force'. The exercise of power-over does not always have to be negative. State legislation to control the spread of diseases, to impose fines for unhealthy behaviour such as smoking in a public place or even to redistribute market income to prevent poverty are all examples of what we consider 'healthy' power-over. Power-over can take different forms and has three functionally distinct operations: dominance, or the direct power to control people's choices, usually by force or its threat; exploitation, or the indirect power to control people's choices through economic relations, in which those who control capital (primarily money) also have control over those who do not and hegemony, or the ability of a dominant group to control the actions and behaviours of others by intense persuasion (Wrong, 1988).

Power-with describes a different set of social relationships, in which power-over is deliberately used to increase other people's power-from-within, rather than to dominate or exploit them. Power-over transforms to power-with only when it has effectively reached its end, when the submissive person in the relationship has accrued enough power-from-within to exercise his or her own choices and decisions. Western feminist theory supports the concept of power-with in that the greater the development of each individual the more able, effective and less dependent on others they become (Swift and Levin, 1987). Feminist theory holds that even in the most male-dominated, power-over societies, women have power, their power-from-within. Once one has accepted this, the argument that people can both have and lack power-over in society can be seen to contain an important insight. Power-over becomes a decentred notion: A person may hold a great deal of authority in one aspect of their life but possess very little in other aspects of their life. An immigrant may hold the position of a leader within their own *community*, but within the work place in their adopted country may have only a low-paying menial job with little responsibility and be considered a second-class citizen by some of their colleagues (Laverack, 2004).

Starhawk (1990, p. 10) identifies the source of power-with as '...the willingness of others to listen to our ideas'. The person with the power-over chooses not to command or exert control, but to suggest and to begin a discussion that will increase the other's sense of power-from-within. With respect to some facets of community members' lives, health promotion practitioners may have knowledge and resources useful to them and may give priority to communities that are relatively powerless. Rather than a simple transfer of resources and information, then, the professional relationship involves an offering of advice and strategies to develop both the psychological *empowerment* (self-esteem and self-confidence) of individuals and the collective empowerment of communities.

KEY TEXTS
- Laverack, G. (2004) *Health Promotion Practice: Power and Empowerment* (London: Sage Publications)
- Laverack, G. (2009) *Public Health: Power, Empowerment & Professional Practice*. 2nd edn (Basingstoke: Palgrave Macmillan)
- Scott, J. (2001) *Power* (Cambridge, UK: Polity Press)

powerlessness

SEE ALSO **empowerment; hegemonic power; individualism and health; networks; power; self-help groups**

Powerlessness, or the absence of *power*, whether imagined or real is a concept with the expectancy that the behaviour of a person or group cannot determine the outcomes they seek (Kieffer, 1984).

Powerlessness is viewed as a continuous interaction between the person and his/her environment. It combines an attitude of self-blame, a sense of generalized distrust, a feeling of alienation from resources for social influence, an experience of disenfranchisement and economic vulnerability and a sense of hopelessness in sociopolitical struggle (Kieffer, 1984). Learned helplessness is a similar psychological construct that emerged from Martin Seligman's animal research in the 1960s. Dogs were subjected to inescapable electric shocks. When the barrier preventing their escape from these shocks was removed, the dogs continued to withstand them anyway and did not seek escape. Even if they accidentally avoided the shocks, they did not internalize this learning and continued to endure subsequent shocks. They had resigned themselves to their fate; they had 'learned helplessness'. The dogs, however, did 're-learn' how to escape after repeated 'teachings' by the researchers, in which the dogs were pushed, pulled or prodded away from the area being shocked. Martin Seligman has now coined another term, 'learned optimism', to encompass the dynamic of learning how to develop positive self-images (Peterson, Maier and Seligman, 1995). Michael Lerner (1986), a political scientist and psychotherapist, argues that a similar phenomenon occurs with persons living in risk conditions. He named this process 'surplus powerlessness', a surplus created by, but distinct from, external or objective conditions of powerlessness. Individuals internalize powerlessness and this creates a potent psychological barrier to empowering action or other activities that meet their real needs. They accept aspects of their world that are self-destructive to their own wellbeing, thinking that these are unalterable features of what they take to be 'reality' (Lerner, 1986). Cynically, this has also been termed the 'apathy of the poor'.

Powerlessness may also be viewed as a result of the passive acceptance of oppressive cultural 'givens', or the surrender to a 'culture of silence' (Freire, 1973). Paulo Freire believed that the individual becomes powerless in assuming the role of 'object' acted upon by the environment, rather than the 'subject' acting in and on the world. As such, the individual alienates himself/herself from participation in the construction of social reality (Wallerstein, 1992). The powerless often experience little *leverage* on the events and conditions that impinge on their existence, either directly or through access to resources that guarantee survival, decrease discomfort and enable change and betterment in one's life (Kroeker, 1995). Radical relativism that maintains that the only 'true' reality is the unique experience of the individual. Intersubjectivity is a concept used to overcome the limitations of radical relativism. It claims that any given person's understanding of the world is unique, but because it is constructed from a field of more or less common social meanings and experiences, communication between people is possible. In other words, the meanings we create of our own experiences, for example, of health, overlap sufficiently so that we can communicate and share these with others. Social *networks* and *self-help groups* are therefore important health promotion strategies to help others to overcome the constraints of perceived powerlessness.

Rather than begin their work from the perspective that their clients who are, in general terms, 'relatively' economically and politically powerless, health promotion practitioners need to look for, and work from, areas in peoples' lives in which they are 'relatively' powerful. This can mean areas in people's lives where they have some power-over or power-from within and to assist individuals to organize themselves both individually and collectively to increase their exercise of power-over the influences on their lives and health, including its determinants.

KEY TEXTS

- Laverack, G. (2004) *Health Promotion Practice: Power and Empowerment* (London: Sage Publications)
- Peterson, C., Maier, S. and Seligman, M. (1995) *Learned Helplessness: A Theory for the Age of Personal Control* (New York: Oxford University Press)
- Scott, J. (2001) *Power* (Cambridge, UK: Polity Press)

pressure groups

SEE ALSO advocacy; civil society; empowerment; health activism; networks; social movements

Pressure groups are commonly formed on the basis of the interests of their members such as professional or community-based organizations and are based on a particular cause. The common aim of pressure groups is to change the opinions and attitudes of society and to influence the policy-making process, but not to govern (Young and Everritt, 2004).

The aforementioned description of a pressure group can also apply to *advocacy* and interest groups but differs from social movements that are able to be representative of an ideology of greater equity, with broader social *networks*. There is an important distinction to be made between pressure groups that are supported by an outside agent such as a health service employer, and those that are independent and are formed by its members, for the benefit of its members. 'Health consumer groups', for example, are voluntary organizations that promote and represent the interests of the users or carers of health services, usually formed at a national level (Allsop, Jones and Baggott, 2004). These groups cover a range of health conditions including heart disease, mental health and maternal and child health. Health consumer groups are mostly charitable organizations and are focussed on one particular policy issue choosing to use tactics such as sharing information, providing support services for its members, *lobbying* and online resources. The Patient UK website, for example, provides links to more than 1,800 patient support groups covering a range of conditions as well as forums through which people can support each other and can create new pressure groups on health-related issues (Patient UK, 2012).

Another practical example of a pressure group was the national campaign to fund the use of Herceptin® more widely to treat breast cancer in the United Kingdom. Herceptin® works by interfering with the way breast cancer cells divide and grow. The minimum cost to pay for the treatment is well beyond the means of most women who have breast cancer. The high cost of Herceptin® owes partly not only to the expense of research leading to its development, but also to the extension of intellectual property rights under international trade treaties that prevents the manufacture of cheaper 'generic' equivalents. However, the National Health Service Trusts refused to fund the drug until it was licensed for use in the early stages of the condition because of safety concerns and the absence of a product licence for the drug's use in the United Kingdom. The Trusts indicated that they would wait for a published decision from the National Institute of Health and Clinical Excellence (NICE). This decision outraged many women who then established local pressure groups to organize and mobilize themselves to try and bring about a change in the decision made by local trusts. Ordinary women organized actions such as local demonstrations outside hospitals, petitions, sit-in protests and wrote to their Member of Parliament. The women established a website to support other women and embarked on an aggressive publicity campaign against the government. As a direct result of the pressure group, the NICE was put under pressure to make a quick decision on the use of Herceptin®. Eventually, the success of a high-profile court case ensured that Herceptin® was approved for use on the National Health Service. This was largely because of the determined action of women at the national level to have a wider influence on the distribution of Herceptin® to others (Boseley, 2006).

The risk when working with pressure groups is that they simply become actors in a process that actually enhances the legitimacy of government policy or corporate interests as they purse their own broader agenda. This is because pressure groups are usually short term and have little influence and resources, even if they are able to form some kind of an alliance or partnership with others that share their concerns (Allsop, Jones and Baggott, 2004).

KEY TEXTS
- Allsop, J., Jones, K. and Baggott, R. (2004) 'Health Consumer Groups in the UK: A New Social Movement', *Sociology of Health & Illness*, 26 (6): pp. 737–756
- Laverack, G. (2013) *Health Activism: Foundations and Strategies* (London: Sage Publications), Chapter 8
- Watts, D. (2007) *Pressure Groups* (Edinburgh: Edinburgh University Press)

primary health care

SEE ALSO **community-based intervention; declarations and statements; disease prevention; public health**

Primary health care is essential health care made accessible at a cost a country and/or *community* can afford, with methods that are practical, scientifically sound and socially acceptable (WHO, 1978).

The declaration of Alma Ata was adopted at the international conference on primary health care in September 1978 (WHO, 1978) and emphasized the importance of prevention, participation and the need for social and political action to address poor health. It was the first international conference underlining the importance of primary health care and was subsequently accepted by the member states of the WHO as key to achieving 'health for all'.

Recently, the WHO has updated its interpretation of primary health care as simply an ultimate goal of better health for all and in so doing identified five key elements to achieving that goal:

1. reducing exclusion and social disparities in health (universal coverage reforms);
2. organizing health services around people's needs and expectations (service delivery reforms);

3. integrating health into all sectors (public policy reforms);
4. pursuing collaborative models of policy dialogue (*leadership* reforms) and
5. increasing stakeholder participation (WHO, 2008a).

As a set of activities, primary health care should include at the very least *health education* for the whole community on preventing and controlling local health problems. In addition, there is also scope for health promotion through the day-to-day contact between primary health care personnel and individuals in their community. Through health education with clients, and *advocacy* on behalf of their community, primary health care personnel are well placed both to support individual needs and to influence the policies and programmes that affect the health of the community (WHO, 1998). Other essential activities include the promotion of food and proper nutrition; sufficient safe water and basic sanitation; maternal and child health care, family planning, immunization, the appropriate treatment of common diseases and injuries and the provision of essential drugs. Primary health care is expected to contribute to many of the prerequisites for health including adequate economic resources, food and shelter, a stable eco-system and a sustainable resource use.

KEY TEXTS
- Greenhalgh, T. (2007) *Primary Health Care: Theory and Practice* (London: BMJ Books)
- Jirojwong, S. and Liamputtong, P. (eds) (2009) *Population Health, Communities and Health Promotion* (Oxford: Oxford University Press), Chapter 2
- World Health Organization (2008a) *The World Health Report: Primary Health Care* (Now more than ever) (Geneva: World Health Organization)

public health

SEE ALSO **global health; health protection; healthy public policy; primary health care**

Public health is an approach that aims to promote health, prevent disease, treat illnesses, prolong valued life, care for the infirm and to provide health services. Traditionally, such goals have been used to curb the spread of infectious diseases and to protect the wellbeing of the general population, while others see a much greater role in regulation and reducing inequalities in health (Baggott, 2010).

The range of public health goals means that the term is used to cover a number of specialist areas including health promotion. Not surprisingly, public health remains a contested and sometimes contradictory term given the competing perspectives, priorities and services that it claims to deliver. The early public health movement focussed on the reduction in mortality and morbidity from communicable diseases through key measures such as improving sanitation and bacteriological control. Later, in the twentieth century, public health has focussed on addressing non-communicable diseases through measures such as changing an individual's lifestyle, and reducing risk conditions. Globalization, economic, political and environmental conditions have had a significant impact on the health of populations. Public health was expected to reach for population-wide health improvement across borders and to reduce the causes of health inequalities that were outside the control of individuals. This evolved as the field of *population health* operating at international, national and state levels (Jirojwong and Liamputtong, 2009). The goal of population health is to maintain and improve the health of the entire population, and to reduce inequalities in health between population groups. Public health, on the other hand, aims to reduce disease and maintain and promote the health of a population (WHO, 2004).

The different interests within public health help to shape what it looks like and the directions it takes as a professional practice by the need to compete for limited resources, the control over decisions and the development of national policies. Public health also involves 'communities' and incorporates methods that connect collective action to the broader aims of political influence (Laverack, 2009). As a profession, public health is professionally driven and largely controlled by government departments, private sector agencies or NGOs. These people are employed as 'professionals' to engage in programmes designed to improve or maintain the health of individuals, groups and communities (Turner and Samson, 1995). Public health therefore entails some *power* relationship between its different stakeholders, primarily between practitioners and their clients. Practitioners are employed to deliver information, resources and services and are often seen as an outside agent to the people who are their clients. The term 'clients' covers the range of people who act as the recipients of the information, resources and services being delivered to promote health.

In practice, public health still belongs primarily to people employed in the health sector, in the sense that it provides these workers with some conceptual models, professional legitimacy and resources. These people may be titled 'health promoters' or 'health communicators', while many more who look to the idea of public health occupy jobs such as health visitors, nurses, *health protection* and environmental health officers.

KEY TEXTS

- Baggott, R. (2010) *Public Health: Policy and Politics.* 2nd edn (Basingstoke: Palgrave Macmillan)
- Baum, F. (2008) *The New Public Health.* 3rd edn (Australia and New Zealand: Oxford Higher Education)
- Hanlon, P. *et al.* (2012) *The Future Public Health* (Maidenhead: Open University Press)
- Jirojwong, S. and Liamputtong, P. (eds) (2009) *Population Health, Communities and Health Promotion* (Oxford: Oxford University Press)

r

risk factors

SEE ALSO behaviour change communication; determinants of health; disease prevention; lifestyle approach; networks; power

Risk factors refer to social, economic or biological status, behaviours or environments that are associated with or cause increased susceptibility to a specific disease, ill health or injury. Once risk factors have been identified, they can become the entry point or focus for health promotion strategies and actions (WHO, 1998, p. 18).

The existence of risk factors in, for example, living and working conditions can increase poor health and are unequally distributed and can also change over time. Decades ago, the poor died more frequently than the rich from communicable diseases; today, they also die more frequently than the rich from non-communicable diseases such as heart disease and certain forms of cancer (Laverack, 2004).

Psychosocial risk factors describe individual cognitive or emotional states (such as self-esteem or self-blame), which are often reactions to risk conditions and which also influence our desire and ability to create *social networks*. The stress created by economic insecurity and structural inequality becomes physical pathology, and might be described as follows: People living in risk conditions experience distress with the unfairness of their situation (their low status on some hierarchy of *power* or authority, indicated in part by wealth) and internalize this unfairness as aspects of their own 'badness' or 'failure'. This internalization adds to their distress, if not also to their loss of meaning and purpose, with measurable effects on their bodies, or physiological risk factors. This situation is more likely when the dominant social discourse on success is competitiveness, individualism and meritocracy, where people are presumed to succeed or fail purely on the basis of their own initiative or ability (Lerner, 1986).

People who live in risk conditions, and internalize this as psychosocial risk factors, are also more likely to have unhealthier lifestyles, or associated behavioural risk factors, for example, smoking and alcohol consumption, which can serve as stress-coping 'rewards'. Even if people living in poor conditions do manage to change their unhealthy behaviours, without any change in their risk conditions, their self-reported health can actually worsen (Blaxter, 2010). Health behaviours can be distinguished from risk behaviours, which are associated with increased susceptibility to a specific cause of ill-health. Health behaviours and risk behaviours are often related in clusters in a more complex pattern of behaviours referred to as 'lifestyles'. People caught in this cycle of risk conditions and risk factors experience less social support and greater isolation and are often less likely to be active in *community* groups or processes concerned with improving risk conditions in the first place (Auslander, 1988). This then reinforces their sense of isolation and self-blame, reinforcing the experience of disease or a lack of wellbeing.

Health promotion professionals may begin their work with an individual or a group around a physiological, behavioural or psychosocial risk factor, or around a risk condition. However, they must strip the pathways of health determinants back to their 'risk conditions'; otherwise, they will forever be treating the symptoms and never preventing the cause. The task is to locate these disease and behavioural risks in their psychosocial and socio-environmental contexts, for example, *powerlessness*, poverty and isolation, and to recognize these contexts as independent health risks in their own right.

KEY TEXTS
- Blaxter, M. (2010) *Health*. 2nd edn (Oxford: Polity Press)
- Naidoo, J. and Wills, J. (2009) *Foundations for Health Promotion*. 3rd edn (Edinburgh: Bailliere and Tindall), Chapter 3

S

salutogenesis

SEE ALSO empowerment; health literacy; power; self-help groups

Salutogenesis describes an approach focusing on factors that support human *health and wellbeing*, rather than on factors that cause disease. More specifically, the salutogenic approach is concerned with the relationship between health, stress and coping (Antonovsky, 1979).

The term salutogenesis was developed by the American medical sociologist Aaron Antonovsky. His theories rejected the traditional medical-approach dichotomy separating health and illness and instead described the relationship as a health-ease versus dis-ease continuum (Antonovsky, 1979). The word salutogenesis is derived from the Latin *salus* (health) and the Greek *genesis* (origin). Antonovsky developed the term from his studies of how people manage stress and stay well and (http://en.wikipedia.org/wiki/Salutogenesis – cite_note-unravelingthemystery1987–2) observed that while stress was ubiquitous, not all individuals had negative health outcomes. Instead, some people achieved health despite their exposure to potentially disabling stress factors (Antonovsky, 1987). In his theory, whether a stress factor was pathogenic, neutral or salutary depended on what he called generalized resistance resources (GRRs). A GRR is any coping resource that is effective in avoiding or combating a range of psychosocial stressors: resources such as money, ego-strength and social support.

Antonovsky's formulation was that the GRRs enabled individuals to make sense of and manage events. He argued that over time, in response to positive experiences provided by the successful use of different GRRs, an individual would develop an attitude that was in itself the essential tool for coping (Antonovsky, 1979). The sense of coherence (SOC) is a theoretical formulation that provides a central explanation for the role of stress in human functioning. Antonovsky defined SOC as

> a global orientation that expresses the extent to which one has a pervasive, enduring though dynamic feeling of confidence that (1) the stimuli deriving from one's internal and external environments in the course of living are structured, predictable and explicable; (2) the resources are available to one to meet the demands posed by these stimuli and (3) these demands are challenges, worthy of investment and engagement. (Antonovsky, 1979, p. 123)

In comparison with concepts like coping or resilience (where the conditions and mechanisms are more rigid and contextual), salutogenesis has its strength in adaptability and universal use and as a life orientation always focusing on problem solving.

In Antonovsky's formulation, the SOC has three components:

1. **Comprehensibility:** A belief that things happen in an orderly and predictable manner and a sense that you can understand events in your life and reasonably predict what will happen in the future.
2. **Manageability:** A belief that you have the skills or ability, the support, the help or the resources necessary to take care of things, and that things are manageable and within your control.
3. **Meaningfulness:** A belief that things in life are interesting and a source of satisfaction, that things are really worth it and that there is good reason or purpose to care about what happens.

According to Antonovsky, the third element is the most important. If a person believes there is no reason to persist and survive and confront challenges, if they have no sense of meaning, then they will have no motivation to comprehend and manage events. The essential argument is that salutogenesis depends on experiencing a strong SOC and that this can lead to positive health outcomes. The life orientation questionnaire is the original name of the instrument to measure SOC and consists of 29 items and a shorter version of 13 items with several alternative instruments available. The SOC questionnaire can be used to measure people's ability to maintain health despite stress, although its efficacy has not been fully verified (Lindstrom and Eriksson, 2005).

KEY TEXTS

- Antonovsky, A. (1979) *Health, Stress and Coping* (San Francisco, CA: Jossey-Bass)
- Lindström, B. and Eriksson, M. (2010) 'The Hitchhiker's Guide to Salutogenesis: Salutogenic Pathways to Health Promotion', *Fokhalsan Health Promotion Research Report 2* (Helsinki: Finland)

screening

SEE ALSO **disease prevention; lifespan approach; lifestyle approach; primary health care; public health; risk factors**

Screening interventions are designed to identify disease early, thus enabling prevention management and treatment to reduce mortality from both communicable and chronic diseases including breast, prostate and cervical cancer, diabetes and osteoporosis (Raffle and Muir Gray, 2007).

Mass screening covers a whole population or a subgroup, irrespective of the risk status of the individual. High risk or selective screening is conducted among individuals of a risk populations. The selection of screening tests for an individual depends on age, sex, family history and *risk factors* for certain diseases. Multiphasic screening is the application of two or more screening tests to a large population at one time instead of carrying out separate screening for single diseases (Raffle and Muir Gray, 2007).

Health promotion plays an important role in the delivery of preventive health interventions that may follow screening including the following:

- Chronic *disease prevention* interventions focus on changing people's behaviour so that they adopt a healthier lifestyle through, for example, regular exercise, good nutrition, smoking cessation and the moderate intake of alcohol.
- Communicable disease prevention interventions promote behaviour change to combat, for example, the spread of sexually transmitted diseases through condom use or a drug regime to combat the spread of tuberculosis.

However, the tests used in screening may be incorrect by showing positive for those without disease, called a false positive, or negative for people who have the condition, called a false negative. Screening may also identify abnormalities that would not normally be a problem for the person, for example, for some forms of prostrate cancer. Over-diagnosis can also make a screening programme look successful by finding abnormalities, even though they are sometimes harmless, and are counted as 'lives saved' by the screening, rather than as healthy people with a manageable condition (Raffle and Muir Gray, 2007).

KEY TEXTS
- Raffle, A.E. and Muir Gray, J.A. (2007) *Screening: Evidence and Practice* (Oxford: Oxford University Press)
- UK Screening Portal (2013) 'UK National Screening Committee'. http://www.screening.nhs.uk/ [accessed 27/2/2013]

self-help groups

SEE ALSO civil society; empowerment; needs assessment; patient empowerment; pressure groups

Self-help groups organize around a specific problem such as 'Weight Watchers'. Group members have a shared knowledge and interest in the problem, are supportive to one another and are often managed by the participants their own activities (Laverack, 2009, p. 70).

Self-help, or self-improvement, is a self-guided improvement, economically, intellectually or emotionally, often with a psycho-social basis. Self-help often utilizes support groups, either face to face or through the internet that provide friendship, emotional support, experiential knowledge, meaningful roles and a greater sense of belonging. Self-help groups can be used for health promotion interventions to learn and about health problems and to gain specific skills and to provide peer support. The involvement in, and the development of, small groups by concerned individuals is also an important part of health promotion because they are often the start of collective action. Self-help groups can progress onto become *advocacy* and *pressure groups*. This locale provides an opportunity for the practitioner to assist the individual to develop stronger social support and to mobilize the resources necessary to support action.

Examples of other self-help health groups include the following:

1. *Community* health groups usually come together for a short period of time to campaign on a specific issue, for example, better facilities for socially excluded groups such as the elderly.
2. Community development health projects such as neighbourhood-based projects set up to address issues of local concern such as poor housing, and with an appointed and paid government community worker.

Self-help groups bring people together and help them to identify issues that they feel are important to them. *Needs assessment* skills are necessary to be able to identify the common problems of their members, solutions to the problems and actions to resolve the problems. When these skills do not exist or are weak, the role of the practitioner is to assist the group to make an assessment of its own needs. Self-help and other groups build their capacity through the achievement of realistic goals as a part of forward planning. In one study, successful groups were found to have a number of key characteristics including a membership of elected representatives, they met on a regular basis, a structure (chairperson, secretary and core members), keeping records and financial accounts, and they were able to identify and resolve conflicts quickly (Jones and Laverack, 2003).

Self-help groups often have limited resources, and because of their small size, the inclusion in the policy process can actually lead to them being absorbed unless they are able to grow and develop into broader community-based organizations (Allsop, Jones and Baggott, 2004). The challenge for the health promoter is to enable people to move forward from individual issues, to be included in small groups and later in community-based organizations and partnerships. This allows people to have greater capacity to work with others who share the same concerns and with whom they can take the necessary actions to resolve their problems.

KEY TEXTS

- Allsop, J., Jones, K. and Baggott, R. (2004) 'Health Consumer Groups in the UK: A New Social Movement', *Sociology of Health and Illness*, 26 (6): pp. 737–756

- Farris Kurtz, L. (1997) *Self-Help and Support Groups: A Handbook for the Practitioner* (London: Sage Publications)
- Watts, D. (2007) *Pressure Groups* (Edinburgh: Edinburgh University Press)

settings

SEE ALSO **approaches; civil society; healthy public policy; public health; risk factors**

A setting is a place or social context in which people engage in daily activities and in which environmental, organizational and personal factors interact to affect *health and wellbeing* (WHO, 1998, p. 19).

Settings can normally be identified as having physical boundaries, a range of people with defined roles and an organizational structure. Examples of settings include schools, workplaces, hospitals and prisons. Settings can be used to promote health by reaching people who work in them, using them to gain access to services, through the interaction of different settings with the wider *community*, through change to the physical environment or an organizational structure. A settings approach to health promotion therefore aims to make systematic changes to the whole environment and not just as a channel through which to access and educate people (Naidoo and Wills, 2009) and can also extend to a 'virtual setting' such as through the use of social media and the internet.

A healthy settings approach can be long term and complex and comprised of many interventions to create supportive environments and *healthy public policy*. A settings approach has unique characteristics including an ecological model of health promotion, a focus on health and wellbeing and the perspective that settings are complex systems and interact with their environment and the organizations within it (Dooris, 2006).

The complexity of the settings approach has made the *evaluation* of its effectiveness problematic, although the *evidence base* for its use in, for example, hospitals, schools, workplaces cities and islands is growing. These particular settings are discussed in more detail below.

A health promoting hospital does not only provide high-quality comprehensive medical and nursing services, but also develop a corporate identity that embraces the aims of health promotion and develop a health promoting organizational structure, culture and physical environment (WHO/EURO, 1991). Health promoting hospitals take a holistic approach to promote the health of their patients, their staff and the population in the community they are located in. The concept of health promoting hospitals started in 1988 and a professional network has developed through the European office of the WHO to promote the approach including in other health care settings. The objectives of this network are to change the culture of hospital care towards interdisciplinary working, transparent decision making and with active involvement of patients and partners; to evaluate health promotion activities in the health care setting and to incorporate standards and indicators for health promotion in existing quality management systems.

Health promoting schools are characterized as constantly strengthening their capacity as a healthy setting for living, learning and working. To achieve this goal, a health promoting school fosters health and learning with all the measures at its disposal. It engages health and education officials, teachers, teachers' unions, students, parents, health providers and community leaders in efforts to make the school a healthy place. A healthy environment is provided through school *health education* and health services, school/community projects and outreach, nutrition and food safety, physical education and recreation and counselling. The school implements policies and practices that respect an individual's wellbeing and dignity as well as the health of school personnel, families and community members. Another important aspect is working with local leaders to help them understand how the community contributes to, or undermines, the health and education of its pupils (WHO, 1997a). WHO's Global School Health Initiative aims at helping all schools to be health promoting through research and capacity building and supports international, national and local *networks*.

The concept of the health promoting workplace developed out of the concept of workplace health promotion that was prominent in the 1970s. In the early stages of its evolution, health promotion activities in the workplace tended to focus on a single illness or on changing a particular lifestyle habit or the behaviour of individual workers. Workplace health promotion activities were dominated by 'wellness' programmes targeting identified *risk factors* associated with employee health. Interventions included health *screening*, stress management courses, nutritional choices in canteens, exercise activities and health information seminars. However, the majority of wellness programmes focused on individual behaviour modification without regard to the broader socio-economic, environmental and organizational influences on workers' health. In the 1990s, workplace health promotion reoriented to be more holistic and to address both individual risk factors and broader organizational and environmental issues. For example, instead of using the workplace as a convenient location to change individual behaviours, workplace health promotion involved both workers and management collectively, endeavouring to change the workplace into a health promoting setting (Chu *et al.*, 2000).

WHO has called for the development of a comprehensive approach towards the promotion of the health of all working populations. This approach is based on four fundamental complementary principles: health promotion, occupational health and safety, human resource management and sustainable development. Fundamental to this approach are multi-sectoral partnerships and the involvement and co-operation of the key actors not only from within a specific workplace but also from all areas that influence working (WHO, 1997). Workplace health also took on renewed impetus after the 60th World Health Assembly in 2007, which endorsed the WHO Global Plan of Action on Workers' Health 2008–2017. The Plan stipulates the need to address all aspects of workers' health, including primary prevention of occupational hazards, protection and promotion of health at work and improved response from health systems to workers' health. To promote workers' health, the workplace should not be detrimental to health and wellbeing, priority should be given to the prevention of occupational health hazards and an integrated response to the specific health needs of working populations should encompass all components of health systems and all of the workplace community.

A healthy city is one 'that is continually creating and improving physical and social environments and expanding community resources which enable people to mutually support each other in performing all the functions of life and to their maximum potential' (WHO, 1998, p. 13). The healthy city programme is a long-term international development initiative that aims to place health high on the agendas of decision makers and to promote comprehensive local strategies for *health protection* and sustainable development. The healthy city concept depends not on current health infrastructure, but rather on a commitment to improve a city's environs and a willingness to forge the necessary connections in political, economic and social arenas. It includes community participation and *empowerment*, inter-sectoral partnerships and participant equity and is evolving to encompass other forms of settlement including healthy villages and municipalities.

The first ministerial meeting of health for the Pacific Islands was convened in Fiji in 1995, and resulted in the Yanuca Island Declaration on Health in the Pacific in the twenty-first century. Healthy Islands are places where children are nurtured in body and mind, environments invite learning and leisure, people work and age in dignity and ecological balance is a source of pride. The Yanuca Declaration has since become an inter-regional source of reference for 'Healthy Islands' programmes throughout the world. A healthy island is defined as the one that is committed to and involved in a process of achieving better health and quality of life for its people, and healthier physical and social environments in the context of *sustainable development* (WHO, 1998, p. 13). To achieve this, some island countries have focused on the control of specific diseases or health problems, such as malaria control in the Solomon Islands and environmental health and health promotion initiatives in the Fiji Islands (WHO Regional Office for the Western Pacific, 1995).

Other settings are becoming increasingly important as they provide opportunities for health promoters to reach marginalized groups, for example, in prisons. The concept of a 'health promoting prison' developed in the 1990s and has since been guided by the WHO. This concept attempts to include all aspects of prison life including the needs of the individual, the organizational and physical environment. Prisoners are socially excluded, often have poor educational backgrounds, low self-esteem, have suffered from homelessness and poor employment opportunities and have had stressful relationships with others in society, including with their own family members. The prevalence of illness, for example, mental health, is higher than in the wider community and a health promotion approach, as well as a *disease prevention* approach, is an essential part of work in prison settings (Dixey *et al.*, 2013, p. 114).

KEY TEXTS

- Dooris, M. (2006) 'Healthy Settings: Challenges to Generating Evidence of Effectiveness', *Health Promotion International*, 21 (1): pp. 55–65
- Naidoo, J. and Wills, J. (2009) *Foundations for Health Promotion.* 3rd edn, Part 3 (Edinburgh: Bailliere and Tindall)
- Scriven, A. and Hodgins, M. (2011) *Health Promotion Settings: Principles and Practice* (London: Sage Publications)

social epidemiology

SEE lay epidemiology

social justice

SEE ALSO civil society; determinants of health; gender and health; political activity; power; powerlessness

Social justice can be defined as justice that is exercised within a society. A socially just society is one based on the principles of equality, equity and solidarity and one that both values and practices human rights as well as recognizing the dignity of every human being (Zajda, Majhanovich and Rust, 2006).

Two major theories on social justice differ in their emphasis on means or ends: equality of opportunity or equality of outcome. The first, and politically dominant, theory holds to the importance of ensuring that everyone 'plays by the same rules'; there is no discrimination. Fairness is judged by equality in process. The second, and politically challenging, theory holds to the importance of ensuring that rules work to minimize preventable differences in outcomes between the stakeholders. It discriminates positively in favour of those groups who start life with fewer resources since equal rules for unequal stakeholders will always produce unequal results. While fairness in process is important, concerns with preventable differences in health outcomes aligns itself ethically more closely to the second theory of justice (Laverack, 2004). Equity, as applied to health, is a normative judgment of what is fair. It differs from equality, a measure of sameness, although the terms are often used interchangeably, where health inequality has become synonymous with health inequity (Braveman and Gruskin, 2003).

A health inequity is a difference (an inequality) in health (however measured) that is significant in size and number of people affected, preventable through policy or other intervention and not an effect of freely chosen risk. A major concern is social inequities that reside in the structures of society, creating systematic differences in health outcomes between different population groups such as gender differences that arise from patriarchal norms or discrimination, class differences that arise from inequalities in wealth and *power* and ownership/control of capital.

There are four useful and empirically supported ways in which to approach how social injustice and societal structures create health inequities:

1. **Social stratification:** where people are located in a social gradient (by economic, gender and racial status).
2. **Differential exposure:** to risks or hazards in the workplace, the *community*, the broader social and physical environments; the response to which is influenced by pre-existing.
3. **Differential vulnerability:** this increases the likelihood of morbidity or mortality when exposed to risks or hazards.
4. **Differential consequences:** both in terms of access to remedial health or other social services, length of time recovering from illness and the impact of illness on their position in a social gradient (Diderichsen, Evans and Whitehead, 2001).

The degree of stratification and differential exposure, vulnerability and consequences is very much a function of economic and political policies. Among high-income countries, those favouring a more 'liberal' (or neo-liberal) political economy have given lower priority to policies aimed at social spending than have social democratic countries, for example, in the Nordic countries (Labonte and Laverack, 2008). Social injustice manifests across *civil society* and reflects unequal differences in the wealth and power of people. Those people who are already disenfranchised are further disadvantaged with respect to their health and freedom (WHO, 2008). Any serious effort to reduce social injustice and health inequities must therefore involve changing the distribution of power within society, empowering individuals and groups to represent strongly and effectively their needs and interests and, in so doing, to challenge and change the unfair distribution of social and material resources.

It is now, more than ever, recognized that the key to addressing social injustice and inequities in health is through the redistribution of power and by transforming unequal power relationships within and between societies. Health inequity in the conditions of daily living is shaped by deep social structures and processes, is systematic and can be enhanced by social norms and government policies that tolerate or actually promote unfair distribution of and access to power, wealth and other necessary social resources (WHO, 2008).

KEY TEXTS
- Cannon, M. and Perkins, J. (2009) *Social Justice Handbook* (Nottingham, UK: IVP Books)
- Capeheart, L. and Milovanovic, D. (2007) *Social Justice: Theories, Issues and Movements* (Biggleswade, UK: Rutgers University Press)
- Zajda, J., Majhanovich, S. and Rust, V. (2006) *Education and Social Justice* (London: Springer)

social marketing

SEE ALSO **behaviour change communication; information, education and communication; health education; health literacy**

Social marketing reflects commercial sector marketing technologies applied to social and health problems that are then resolved by behaviour change (Andreasen, 1995).

Social marketing has been used in a variety of successful *community* health behaviour change projects and has been examined with a wide range of benchmarked successes. Gordon *et al.* (2006), for example, assessed the evidence for social marketing in nutrition and physical activity behaviour change showing increases in knowledge and reasonable efficacy in influencing psychosocial variables. Social marketing has been used by different agencies in the United States to increase fruit and vegetable consumption and to promote breastfeeding. In other countries, social marketing has been used to eliminate leprosy, increase adherence to medication to treat tuberculosis and to promote immunization. VERB™ is a national and multi-cultural social marketing intervention in the United States. The programme encourages young people between the ages of

9 and 13 years to be physically active each day and uses the mass media, advertising, public relations, interpersonal marketing and partnerships with sports-based organizations. This programme has claimed a 34% increase in weekly free-time physical activity sessions among 8.6 million of its target group with pockets of even higher success rates in some community-based projects (Grier and Bryant, 2005).

Social marketing strategies are concerned first with the needs, preferences and social and economic circumstances of the target audience. This information is used to ensure that the most attractive benefits of a product, service or idea are offered and to address any barriers to its acceptance (Maibach, Rothschild and Novelli, 2002). Communicating with the target audience about the relative advantages of what is offered is one element of social marketing as are efforts to address the economic and regulatory environment. The target audience is a specific group of people at which a health promoting message or product is aimed, for example, if the health outcome is to reduce heart disease the communication may be aimed at the spouse, as well as the middle-aged husband. A target audience can be formed of a number of factors and of people of a certain age group, gender and marital status (Kotler, 2000).

Social marketing programmes usually incorporate all or a mix of the following four Ps:

1. create an enticing **product** (i.e., the package of benefits associated with the desired action);
2. minimize the **price** the target audience believes it must pay in the exchange;
3. make the exchange and its opportunities available in **places** that reach the audience and fit its lifestyles;
4. **promote** the exchange opportunity with creativity and through channels and tactics that maximize desired responses.

Despite the popularity and influence of the social marketing approach, many health promotion professionals still have a narrow view of what it is and what it can achieve. Many professionals view social marketing as a simple communication strategy, while others feel that it is too coercive or manipulative and 'blames the victim' rather than addressing underlying environmental and social causes. Social marketing requires considerable planning, expertise and resources to be effective and may therefore be too time consuming and expensive for many health promotion projects. However, success has been achieved by building a social marketing intervention into larger national health promotion programmes and then adapting the approach to fit unique national- or local-level requirements such as targeting cultural preferences (Grier and Bryant, 2005).

KEY TEXTS

- Corcoran, N. (ed) (2013) *Communicating Health: Strategies for Health Promotion.* 2nd edn (London: Sage Publications)
- Lee, N. and Kotler, P. (2011) *Social Marketing: Influencing Behaviours for Good.* 4th edn (London: Sage Publications)
- Weinreich, N. (2010) *Hands-On Social Marketing: A Step by Step Guide to Designing Change for Good.* 2nd edn (London: Sage Publications)

t

theory and models

SEE ALSO approaches; definition; evidence-based practice; healthy public policy; individualism and health

Theory is systematically organized knowledge applicable in a relatively wide variety of circumstances devised to analyse, predict or otherwise explain the nature or behaviour of a specified set of phenomena that could be used as the basis for action (Van Ryn and Heany, 1992).

Health promotion theory originates from the social and behavioural sciences drawing on knowledge from psychology, sociology, management, marketing, *community* development and the political sciences. Health promotion theory includes a broad range of ideas and concepts, many of which have not been fully tested in practice. This has resulted in a more analytical means to develop 'models' for practice that seek to represent simplified versions of reality but do not truly reflect the complexities of social behaviour (Naidoo and Wills, 2009).

A major challenge in health promotion practice is how to apply the correct theory and models (the science) to the appropriate practice context (the art). Health promotion programmes often cover a range of issues, target groups, *settings* and cultural contexts, and in practice, this may necessitate the use of more than one theory or model. In addition, health promotion practitioners are constrained by time, finances and even the level of control that they have over which theory and models they can use in a programme. To make matters more confusing, there are a number of overlapping models for health promotion but with no real consensus on terminology and criteria (Nutbeam, Harris and Wise, 2010).

Implicit in the use of health promotion models is the theoretical framework that explains how and why its different aspects are connected (Naidoo and Wills, 2009). When choosing a theoretical framework to best fit the health promotion problem, it is useful to follow these guidelines:

- Is it simple to understand and logical?
- Does it match everyday observations of the problem?
- Has it been successfully used previously in a similar context?
- Is it supported by the evidence of what works?
- Can it be justified in terms of the resources necessary?
- Can it be measured?

From a practical perspective, Naidoo and Wills (2009, chapter 5) discuss two models of health promotion that use criteria from social policy frameworks and a structural analysis of influences that contribute to inequalities in health. The models also show how health promotion *approaches* can be influenced by political ideology, *power*, personal responsibility and autonomy.

1. The model by Tannahill (Downie, Tannahill and Tannahill, 1996) discusses three overlapping areas that interact to create a process of health promotion: *health education; health protection* and health prevention. The model is popular with health care workers because it helps to explain the scope of work in health promotion. However, it does not explain why a practitioner may choose one approach over another as the three are interrelated, even though in practice they represent three distinct ways of working.
2. The model by Tones and Tilford (2001) is useful because it engages with the core goal of health promotion, enabling people to increase control over their health. The model uses a simple equation that *healthy public policy* plus health education creates health promotion practice. Tones and Tilford's model includes both individual and collective *empowerment* as a means of people creating a healthier environment and lifestyle through the knowledge and skills that they gain from health education.

While it is not possible to fully discuss such a broad subject area in this entry, Nutbeam, Harris and Wise (2010) provide an easily accessible summary of theories and models used in health promotion that include the following:

- Theories that explain individual health behaviour change (the health belief approach, theories of reasoned action, the stages of change approach and the social cognitive theory and models that guide communication for behaviour change (*health literacy* and *social marketing*). These theories use health education and the importance of self-belief in one's ability to change behaviour, the development of personal skills and the importance of perceived norms and social influences on the individual such as the role of family, friends and peer groups.
- Theories on change in community through collective action (diffusion of innovation theory, community organization and capacity building). These theories provide opportunities for *community-based intervention*, empowerment and addressing the broader socio-economic *determinants of health*.
- Theories and models for organizational change and inter-sectoral action.
- Models for the development of *healthy public policy* and health impact assessment.

On a day-to-day basis not all health promotion practitioners have the time or the *competencies* to operate at multiple theoretical levels. While applying the 'art and science' of health promotion does not guarantee a successful programme, the use of theory and models in planning and implementation will increase the chances of it being more effective (Nutbeam, Harris and Wise, 2010). Theories and models can therefore provide a structured, and sometimes *evidence-based practice*, approach to plan and implement health promotion programmes.

KEY TEXTS
- Dixey, R. *et al.* (2013) *Health Promotion: Global Principles and Practice* (Wallingford, Oxfordshire: CAB International), Chapter 1
- Naidoo, J. and Wills, J. (2009) *Foundations for Health Promotion.* 3rd edn (Edinburgh: Bailliere and Tindall), Chapter 5
- Nutbeam, D., Harris, E. and Wise, M. (2010) *Theory in a Nutshell: A Practical Guide to Health Promotion Theories.* 3rd edn (London: McGraw-Hill)
- Sharma, M. and Romas, J.A. (2010) *Theoretical Foundations of Health Education and Health Promotion* (Boston, MA: Jones and Bartlett Learning)

Z

zero and non-zero-sum

SEE ALSO community capacity building; hegemonic power; leverage; power; powerlessness

A zero-sum situation exists when one can only possess x amount of power to the extent that someone else has an absence of an equivalent amount of *power* (Laverack, 2004, p. 34).

Power is often interpreted as a finite entity in which one person, group or organization has influence and mastery over others. Zero-sum power creates a 'win/lose' situation. My power-over you, plus your absence of that power, equals zero (thus the term, 'zero-sum'). I win and you lose. For you to gain power, you must seize it from me. If you can, you win and I lose. It is important to understand that power has to be gained or seized by those who want to achieve it, by raising the position of one person or group, while simultaneously lowering it for another person or group (Laverack, 2004).

Zero-sum power is often used in association with economic or political accounts where power is equated to wealth and income, authority and status and is particularly dominant in Western societies. At any one time, there will be only so much wealth possessed within a society. This distribution and the decision-making authority that goes with it is zero-sum. One has authority or social status by virtue of others not having it. There is a degree of flexibility here, however, since someone may have authority or status in one situation, relative to others, but not in another. At the same time, there are dominant social forms of status or privilege, such as class, gender, education, ethnic background, age and even physical ability or sexual preference, which tend to structure power-over relations in most social situations. For example, an immigrant man may hold the position of a *community* leader or hereditary chief within his own ethnic community, but within his work place have only a low-paying menial job with little responsibility or status.

In the same way, the beneficiaries of a health promotion programme may bring with them a great deal of power in the form of authority and control within their community. These individuals can be an important factor in enabling others to take control of the influences on their lives and health such as using local leaders to manage programmes assisted by 'technical experts' to improve the skills and *competencies* of these individuals. The role of health promotion in this zero-sum construction of power is to assist others to gain power, meaning here more control over resources or decision making that influence their health, from other groups. Within communities, this can become a difficult issue. David Zakus and Catherine Lysack (1998), two Canadian health researchers, argue that health promotion practice that works from a zero-sum construction of power actually increases 'unhealthy' competition between people and decreases 'healthy' community capacity and cohesion. They also suggest that by empowering some at the expense of others in a zero-sum situation, health promoters are helping to break down the ties that hold a community together. However, communities are not homogeneous but by their very nature consist of competing heterogeneous individuals and groups. Health promoters cannot therefore avoid empowering some while not others through the interventions and programmes that they deliver. The point raised by Zakus and Lysack (1998) does help to highlight the ethical and political dilemma of which some groups, at the expense of others, should get priority of the limited resources and assistance from the health promoters. This problem is confounded, however, if the group is unpopular or involved in illegal or unpalatable activities such as drug use or child abuse. The role of the health promoter is to be non-judgmental but to be self-reflecting in their work.

There is another important use of power, one that regard it not as fixed and finite, but as infinite and expanding. This is a 'non-zero-sum' form of power that is 'win/win', since it is based on the idea that if any one person or group gains, everyone else also gains. Knowledge, trust, caring and other aspects of our social relationships with one another are examples of non-zero-sum power. Perhaps unsurprisingly, health promoters often gravitate towards the non-zero-sum formulation. Certainly, much of the discourse of health promotion emphasising ' ... participation, caring, sharing and responsibility to others' addresses the exercise of power in which all people can benefit. Power is no longer seen as a finite commodity, such as wealth, or as the comparative status and authority that this might confer. Rather, the non-zero-sum takes the form of relationship behaviours based on respect, generosity, service to others, a free flow of information and the commitment to the *ethics* of caring and justice. The role of the health promoter in this construction of power is to use these attributes to engender them in others, for example, through mentoring and counselling. This approach also transfers power between people by encouraging individuals to network and to access information by themselves, in part by providing better access to resources, for example, through a website link.

In practice, health promotion simultaneously involves zero-sum and non-zero-sum formulations of power. Power cannot be given but communities can be enabled by health promoters to take power that they need from others. To do this, health promoters must first identify their own power base (access to resources and influence) and to understand how this can be appropriately acted upon to enable others to gain power through their own endeavours. It is the relationship between the programme stakeholders, which is empowering through the development of abilities and opportunities to seize control over the influences on the determinants of their health.

KEY TEXTS

- Labonte, R. (1998) *A Community Development Approach to Health Promotion: A Background Paper on Practice Tensions, Strategic Models and Accountability Edinburgh* (Scotland: Health Education Board for Scotland)
- Laverack, G. (2004) *Health Promotion Practice: Power and Empowerment* (London: Sage Publications)
- Laverack, G. (2009) *Public Health: Power, Empowerment and Professional Practice.* 2nd edn (Basingstoke: Palgrave Macmillan)

references

Abulof, U. (2011) *What Is the Arab Third Estate? The Huffington Post.* http://www.huffingtonpost.com/uriel-abulof/what-is-the-arab-third-es_b_832628.html [accessed 1/5/2011]

Aggleton, P. (1991) *Health* (London: Routledge)

Alchin, T.M. (1992) 'The Health Promotion Foundations: How Successful Are They?' *Working Papers in Economics* # wp. 92/03 (Sydney: University of Western Sydney)

Aldridge, S. and Rigby, S. (2001) *Counselling Skills in Context* (London: Hodder and Stoughton)

Alinsky, S.D. (1972) *Rules for Radical: A Practical Primer for Realistic Radicals* (New York: Vintage Books)

Allmark, P. and Tod, A. (2006) 'How Should Public Health Professionals Engage with Lay Epidemiology?' *Journal of Medical Ethics,* 32: pp. 460–463

Allsop, J., Jones, K. and Baggott, R. (2004) 'Health Consumer Groups in the UK: A New Social Movement', *Sociology of Health and Illness,* 26 (6): pp. 737–756

Anand, S., Fabienne, P. and Sen, A. (2006) *Public Health, Ethics and Equity* (Oxford: Oxford University Press)

Andersen, G.L. and Herr, K.G. (eds) (2007) *Encyclopaedia of Activism and Social Justice* (London: Sage Publications)

Anderson, E., Shepard, M. and Salisbury, C. (2006) '"Taking Off the Suit": Engaging the Community in Primary Health Care Decision-Making', *Health Expectations,* 9: pp. 70–80

Andreasen, A.R. (1995) *Marketing Social Change* (San Francisco, CA: Jossey-Bass)

Antonovsky, A. (1979) *Health, Stress and Coping* (San Francisco, CA: Jossey-Bass)

Antonovsky, A. (1987) *Unraveling the Mystery of Health – How People Manage Stress and Stay Well* (San Francisco, CA: Jossey-Bass)

Appleton, B. and Sijbesma, C. (2005) 'Hygiene Promotion: Thematic Overview Paper 1 (IRC International Water and Sanitation Centre, Delft, The Netherlands)

ASH (2012) 'Action on Smoking and Health', www.ash.org. [accessed 20/1/2012]

Auslander, G. (1988) 'Social Networks and the Functional Health Status of the Poor: A Secondary Analysis of Data from the National Survey of Personal Health Practices and Consequences', *Journal of Community Health*, 13 (4): pp. 1–4

Baggott, R. (2010) *Public Health: Policy and Politics*. 2nd edn (Basinstoke: Palgrave Macmillan)

Baker, S. *et al.* (1991) *The Injury Fact Book* (New York: Oxford University Press)

Bamberger, M., Rugh, J. and Mabry, L. (2006) *Realworld Evaluation: Working under Budget, Time, Data and Political Constraints* (London: Sage Publications)

Banks, K. *et al.* (2010) *SMS Uprising: Mobile Activism in Africa* (Oxford: Fahamu Books and Pambazuka Press)

Barnes, M. (2002) 'User Movements, Community Development and Health Promotion' in L. Adams, M. Amos and J. Munro (eds), *Promoting Health: Politics and Practice* (London: Sage Publications)

Barry, M. *et al.* (2009) 'The Galway Conference Statement: International Collaboration on the Development of Core Competencies for Health Promotion and Health Education', *Global Health Promotion*, 16 (2): pp. 5–11

Bassett, S.F. and Prapavessis, H. (2007) 'Home-Based Physical Therapy Intervention with Adherence-Enhancing Strategies Versus Clinic Based Management for Patients with Ankle Sprains', *Physical Therapy*, 87 (9): pp. 1132–1143

Baum, F. (1997) 'Public Health and Civil Society: Understanding and Valuing the Connection', *Australian and New Zealand Journal of Public Health*, 21 (7): pp. 673–675

Baum, F. (2007) 'Cracking the Nut of Health Equity: Top Down and Bottom Up Pressure for Action on the Social Determinants of Health', *Promotion and Education*, 14 (2): pp. 90–95

Baum, F. (2008) *The New Public Health*. 3rd edn (Oxford: Oxford Higher Education)

Baum, F. (2011) 'From Norm to Eric: Avoiding Lifestyle Drift in Australian Health Policy', *Australian and New Zealand Journal of Public Health*, 35 (5): pp. 404–406

Beckmann Murray, R., Proctor Zentner, J. and Yakimo, R. (2009) *Health Promotion Strategies through the Life Span*. 8th edn (New Jersey: Pearson Education Inc)

Bernier, N. (2007) 'Health Promotion Program Resilience and Policy Trajectories: A Comparison of Three Provinces' in M. O'Neill *et al.* (eds),

Health Promotion in Canada: Critical Perspectives (Toronto: Canadian Scholars' Press Inc.)

Begoray, D.L., Gillis, D. and Rowlands, G. (2012) *Health Literacy in Context: International Perspectives (Public Health in the 21st Century)* (New York: Nova Science Publishers Inc)

Berridge, V. (2007) 'Public Health Activism', *British Medical Journal*, 335: pp. 1310–1312

Biddix, J.P. and Han Woo, P. (2008) 'Online Networks of Student Protest: The Case of the Living Wage Campaign', *New Media and Society*, 10 (6): pp. 871–891

Black, J.M. *et al.* (2009) *Philosophical Foundations of Health Education* (San Francisco, CA: Jossey-Bass)

Blaxter, M. (2010) *Health*. 2nd edn (Oxford: Polity Press)

Block, P. (2009) *Community: The Structure to Belonging* (San Francisco, CA: Berrett-Koehler Publishers)

Bloor, M. and McIntosh, J. (1990) 'Surveillance and Concealment' in S. Cunningham-Burley and N.P. McKeganey (eds), *Readings in Medical Sociology* (New York: Tavistock/Routledge)

Boas, T. and Jordan Gans-Morse, J. (2009) 'Neoliberalism: From New Liberal Philosophy to Anti-Liberal Slogan', *Studies in Comparative International Development*, 44 (2): p. 143

Boseley, S. (2006) 'Herceptin Costs "put other patients at risk"', *Guardian Weekly*, December, p. 8

Boutilier, M. (1993) *The Effectiveness of Community Action in Health Promotion: A Research Perspective* (Toronto: University of Toronto), ParticiACTION. 3.

Braithwaite, R.L., Bianchi, C. and Taylor, S.E. (1994) 'Ethnographic Approach to Community Organisation and Health Empowerment', *Health Empowerment*, 21 (3): pp. 407–416

Brashers, D.E. *et al.* (2002) 'Social Activism, Self-Advocacy and Coping with HIV Illness', *Journal of Social and Personal Relationships*, 19 (1): pp. 113–133

Braveman, P. and Gruskin, S. (2003) 'Defining Equity in Health (Theory and Methods)', *Journal of Epidemiology and Community Health*, 57 (4): p. 254

Brayne, H., Sargeant, L. and Brayne, C. (1998) 'Could Boxing Be Banned? A Legal and Epidemiological Perspective', *British Medical Journal*, 316: pp. 1813–1815

Brown, P. and Zavestoski, S. (2004) 'Social Movements in Health: An Introduction', *Sociology of Health & Illness*, 26 (6): pp. 679–694

Brown, P. *et al.* (2004) 'Embodied Health Movements: Uncharted Territory in Social Movement Research', *Sociology of Health & Illness*, 26 (1): pp. 50–80

Brown, V.A. (1992) 'Health Care Policies, Health Policies or Policies for Health?' in H. Gardner (ed), *Health Policy Development, Implementation and Evaluation in Australia* (Melbourne: Churchill Livingstone)

Bryant, T. (2006). 'Politics, Public Policy and Population Health' in D. Raphael, T. Bryant and M. Rioux (eds), *Staying Alive: Critical Perspectives on Health, Illness, and Health Care* (Toronto: Canadian Scholars' Press)

Butterfoss, D. (2007) *Coalitions and Partnerships in Community Health* (San Francisco, CA: Jossey-Bass)

Cannon, M. and Perkins, J. (2009) *Social Justice Handbook* (Nottingham, UK: IVP Books)

Capeheart, L. and Milovanovic, D. (2007) *Social Justice: Theories, Issues and Movements* (Biggleswade, UK: Rutgers University Press)

Cattan, M. and Tilford, S. (2006) *Mental Health Promotion. A Lifespan Approach* (Maidenhead: Open University Press)

CDC/ATSDR. Committee on Community Engagement (1997) *Principles of Community Engagement* (Atlanta: GA), pp. 62–63

Chartered Institute of Environmental Health (2012) http://www.cieh.org/. [accessed 15/1/2013]

Chemers, M. (1997) *An Integrative Theory of Leadership* (New Jersey: Lawrence Erlbaum Associates)

Christakis, N.A. and Fowler, J.H. (2007) 'The Spread of Obesity in a Large Social Network Over 32 Years', *New England Journal of Medicine,* 357 (4): pp. 370–379

Christoffel, T. and Gallagher, S. (2005) *Injury Prevention and Public Health: Practical Knowledge, Skills and Strategies* (Boston, MA: Jones and Bartlett Learning)

Chu, C. *et al.* (2000) 'Health promoting Workplaces – International Settings Development', *Health Promotion International,* 15 (2): pp. 155–167

The Cochrane Collaboration, http://www.cochrane.org/ [accessed 15/3/2013]

Code Pink (2012) 'Women for Peace', http://www.codepink4peace.org/. [accessed 16/1/2012]

Coleman, P.T. (2000) 'Power and Conflict' in M. Deutsch and P.T. Coleman (eds), *The Handbook of Conflict Resolution: Theory and Practice* (San Francisco, CA: Jossey-Bass)

Collins, J. *et al.* (2004) 'An Evaluation of a "best practices" Musculoskeletal Injury Prevention Program in Nursing Homes', *Injury Prevention,* 10: pp. 206–211

Communication, Education and Participation (1996) 'A Framework and Guide to Action' (WHO (AMRO/PAHO), Washington, USA)

Corcoran, N. (ed) (2013) *Communicating Health: Strategies for Health Promotion.* 2nd edn (London: Sage Publications)

Cornish, F. and Campbell, C. (2009) 'The Social Conditions for Successful Peer Education: A Comparison of Two HIV Prevention Programs Run by Sex Workers in India and South Africa', *American Journal of Community Psychology,* 44 (1–2): pp. 123–135

Courtenay, W. (2011) *Dying to Be Men: Psychosocial, Environmental and Biobehavioural Directions in Promoting the Health of Men and Boys* (London: Routledge)

Craig, J. and Smyth, R. (2002) *The Evidence-Based Practice Manual for Nurses* (Edinburgh: Churchill Livingstone)

Cribb, A. and Duncan, P. (2002) *Health Promotion and Professional Ethics* (Oxford: Blackwell Publishing)

Curtis, V. *et al.* (2001) 'Evidence of Behaviour Change Following a Hygiene Promotion Programme in Burkina Faso', *Bulletin of the World Health Organisation,* 79 (6): pp. 518–527

Cwikel, J.G. (2006) *Social Epidemiology: Strategies for Public Health Activism* (New York: Columbia University Press)

Daly, S. (2007) 'Women's Health Activism' in G.L. Andersen and K.G. Herr (eds), *Encyclopedia of Activism and Social Justice* (London: Sage Publications)

Dana, D. (2000) *Conflict Resolution* (London: McGraw-Hill)

Delanty, G. (2003) *Community* (New York: Routledge)

Dempsey, C., Battel-Kirk, B. and Barry, M. (2011) *The CompHP Core Competencies Framework for Health Promotion Handbook* (Executive Agency for Health and Consumers: Paris, IUHPE)

Diderichsen, F., Evans, T. and Whitehead, M. (2001) 'The Social Basis of Disparities in Health' in M. Whitehead *et al.* (eds), *Challenging Inequities in Health: From Ethics to Action* (New York: Oxford University Press)

Dixey, R. *et al.* (2013) *Health Promotion: Global Principles and Practice* (Wallingford, Oxfordshire: CAB International)

Dooris, M. (2006) 'Healthy Settings: Challenges to Generating Evidence of Effectiveness', *Health Promotion International,* 21 (1): pp. 55–65

Dormandy, E. *et al.* (2002) 'Variation in Uptake of Serum Screening: The Role of Service Delivery', *Prenatal Diagnosis,* 22 (1): pp. 67–69

Downie, R.S., Tannahill, C. and Tannahill, A. (1996) *Health Promotion: Models and Values.* 2nd edn (Oxford: Medical Publications)

Draper, P. (ed) (1991) *Health through Public Policy* (London: Green Print)

Dryden, W. and Feltham, C. (1993) *Brief Counselling: A Practical Guide for Beginning Practitioners.* (Milton Keynes: Open University Press)

Dubriwny, T. (2012) *The Vulnerable Empowered Woman: Feminism, Post Feminism and Women's Health (Critical Issues in Health and Medicine)* (Biggleswade, UK: Rutgers University Press)

Eberly, D. (2008) *The Rise of Global Civil Society: Building Communities and Nations from the Bottom Up* (New York: Encounter books)

Edelman, C. and Mandle, C. (2009) *Health Promotion throughout the Life Span.* 7th edn (New York: Elsevier/Mosby Publishers)

Edwards, M. (2009) *Civil Society.* 2nd edn (Oxford: Polity Press)

Edwards, M. (2011) *The Oxford Handbook of Civil Society* (Oxford: Oxford University Press)

Estonian National Institute for Health Development (ENIHD) (2013) http://www.tai.ee/ [accessed 27/2/2013]

Everson, S.A. *et al.* (1997) 'Interaction of Workplace Demands and Cardiovascular Reactivity in Progression of Carotid Atherosclerosis: Population Based Study', *British Medical Journal,* 314: pp. 553–558

Every Australian Counts (2012) http://everyaustraliancounts.com.au/. [accessed 17/2/2102]

Ewles, L. and Simnett, I. (2009) *Promoting Health. A Practical Guide.* 5th edn (Edinburgh: Bailliere Tindall)

Farris Kurtz, L. (1997) *Self-Help and Support Groups: A Handbook for the Practitioner* (London: Sage Publications)

Fathers4Justice (2012) http://www.fathers-4-justice.org. [accessed 15/1/2013]

Faulkner, M. (2001) 'Empowerment and Disempowerment: Models of Staff/Patient Interaction', *Nursing Times Research,* 6 (6): pp. 936–948

Forsyth, D.R. (2009) *Group Dynamics.* 5th edn (Singapore: Cengage Learning)

Foucault, M. (1979) *Discipline and Punishment: The Birth of the Prison* (Middlesex: Penguin Books)

Fox, S. and Rainie, L. (2001) 'Vital Decisions: How Internet Users Decide What Information to Trust When They or Their Loved Ones are Sick' in J. Hubley and J. Copeman (eds), (2008) *Practical Health Promotion* (Cambridge, UK: Polity Press), p. 182

Frampton, S., Charmel, P. and Plantree, C. (eds) (2008) *Putting Patients First: Best Practice in Patient Centered Care* (San Francisco, CA: Jossey-Bass)

Freire, P. (1973) *Education for Critical Consciousness* (New York: Seabury Press)

Freire, P. (2005) *Education for Critical Consciousness* (New York: Continuum Press)

Friedman, M. (1999) *Consumer Boycotts: Effecting Change through the Marketplace and Media* (New York: Routledge)

Friis, R. (2010) *Essentials of Environmental Health,* 2nd edn (Boston, MA: Jones and Bartlett Learning)

Frusciante, A.K. (2007) 'Leadership, Participatory Democratic' in G.L. Andersen and K.G. Herr (eds), *Encyclopedia of Activism and Social Justice* (London: Sage Publications)

Gallarotti, G. (2011) 'Soft Power: What Is It, Why Is It Important and the Conditions for its Effective Use', *Journal of Political Power*, 4 (1): pp. 25–47

Gangolli, L.V., Duggal, R., Shukla, A. (eds) (2005) *Review of Health Care in India* (Mumbai: CEHAT)

Gauld, R. (2006) 'Health Policy and the Health System' in R. Miller (ed), *New Zealand Government and Politics* (Auckland: Oxford University Press), pp. 525–535.

Gibbon, M., Labonte, R. and Laverack, G. (2002) 'Evaluating Community Capacity', *Health and Social Care in the Community*, 10 (6): pp. 485–491

Gilmore, G. (2011) *Needs and Capacity Assessment for Health Education and Health Promotion*. 4th edn (Boston, MA: Jones and Bartlett Learning)

Glanz, K., Rimer, B. and Viswanath, K. (eds) (2008) *Health Behavior and Health Education: Theory, Research and Practice*. 44th edn (San Francisco, CA: Jossey-Bass)

Glaser, J. and Salzberg, C. (2011) *The Strategic Application of Information Technology in Health Care Organisations* (San Francisco, CA: Jossey Bass)

Godbold, N. and Vaccarella, M. (2012) *Autonomous, Responsible, Alone: The Complexities of Patient empowerment* (Freeland, Oxfordshire: Interdisciplinary Press)

Goodman, R. *et al.* (1998) 'Identifying and Defining the Dimensions of Community Capacity to Provide a Base for Measurement', *Health Education and Behaviour*, 25 (3): pp. 258–278

Gordon, R. *et al.* (2006) 'The Effectiveness of Social Marketing Interventions for Health Improvement: What's the Evidence?' *Public Health*, 120: pp. 1133–1139

Green, J. and South, J. (2006) *Evaluation* (Maidenhead: Open University Press)

Green, J. and Tones, K. (2010) *Health Promotion: Planning and Strategies*. 2nd edn (London: Sage Publications)

Green, L. and Kreuter, M. (2004) *Health Program Planning: An Educational and Ecological Approach*. 4th edn (London: McGraw-Hill)

Greenhalgh, T. (2007) *Primary Health Care: Theory and Practice* (London: BMJ Books)

Grier, S. and Bryant, C. (2005) 'Social Marketing in Public Health', *Annual Review of Public Health*, 26: pp. 319–339

Guba, E.G. (1990) *The Paradigm Dialog* (London: Sage Publications)

Hackett, M. (2007) 'Community Radio and Television' in G.L. Andersen and K.G. Herr (eds), *Encyclopedia of Activism and Social Justice* (London: Sage Publications)

Hager, N. (2009) 'Symposium on Commercial Sponsorship of Psychiatrist Education. Speech to the Royal Australian and New Zealand College of Psychiatrists Conference', *Rotorua*, 16 October 2009

Hancock, T. (1993) 'Health, Human Development and the Community Ecosystem: Three Ecological Models', *Health Promotion International*, 8(1): 41–47

Hanlon, P. *et al.* (2012) *The Future Public Health* (Maidenhead: Open University Press)

Hanson, R.E. (2010) *Mass Communication: Living in a Media World* (Washington: CQ Press)

Haque, N. and Eng, B. (2011) 'Tackling Inequity through a Photo-Voice Project on the Social Determinants of Health: Translating Photo-Voice Evidence to Community Action', *Global Health Promotion*, 18 (1): pp. 16–19

Harnik, R. (2002) *Public Health Communication: Evidence for Behaviour Change* (New York: Routledge)

Hashagen, S. (2002) *Models of Community Engagement* (Scottish Community Development Centre, Edinburgh, UK), pp. 7–8

Hawker, J. *et al.* (2012) *Communicable Disease Control and Health Protection Handbook.* 3rd edn (Chichester: Wiley Blackwell)

Health Promotion Foundations. http://www.hpfoundations.net/

Health Protection Agency (UK) (2013) http://www.hpa.org.uk/. [accessed 15/3/2013]

Holland, S. (2007) *Public Health Ethics* (Cambridge, UK: Polity Press)

Holmes, L. (2008) *Basics of Public Health Core Competencies* (Boston, MA: Jones and Bartlett Learning)

Hubley, J., Copeman, J. and Woodall, J. (2013) *Practical Health Promotion.* 2nd edn (Cambridge, UK: Polity Press)

Hull, J. (1988). 'Not in My Neighborhood', *Time* (Time Inc). http://www.time.com/time/magazine/article/. [accessed 25/1/2011]

Hunt, K. and Emslie, C. (2001) 'Commentary: The Prevention Paradox in Lay Epidemiology – Rose Revisited', *International Journal of Epidemiology*, 30 (3): pp. 442–446

Hunter, D. (2003) *Public Health Policy* (Cambridge, UK: Polity Press)

ILO, UNESCO and WHO. (2004) 'CBR: A Strategy from Rehabilitation, Equalization of Opportunities, Poverty Reduction, and Social Inclusion of People with Disabilities (joint Position Paper) (Geneva: WHO Press)

Improvement Network. (2011) www.tin.nhs.uk/patient-involvement [accessed 10/11/2011]

IRC International Water and Sanitation Centre. (2013) http://www.irc.nl/. [accessed 22/1/2013]

Israel, B.A. *et al.* (1994) 'Health Education and Community Empowerment: Conceptualizing and Measuring Perceptions of Individual, Organisational and Community Control', *Health Education Quarterly*, 21 (2): pp. 149–70

Jackson, T., Mitchell, S. and Wright, M. (1989) 'The Community Development Continuum', *Community Health Studies*, 8 (1): pp. 66–73

Jadad, A. and O'Grady, L. (2008) 'How Should Health Be Defined?' *British Medical Journal*, Editorial. 337: p. a2900

Jirojwong, S. and Liamputtong, P. (eds) (2009) *Population Health, Communities and Health Promotion* (Oxford: Oxford University Press)

Johansen, E. *et al.* (2013) 'What Works and What Does Not: A Discussion of Popular Approaches for the Abandonment of Female Genital Mutilation', *Obstetrics and Gynaecology International*, Advance access ID 348248

Johnson, J. and Breckon, D. (2006) *Managing Health Education and Promotion Programs: Leadership Skills for the 21st Century*. 2nd edn (Boston, MA: Jones and Barlett Publishers)

Jones, A. and Laverack, G. (2003) 'Building Capable Communities within a Sustainable Livelihoods Approach: Experiences from Central Asia', http://www.livelihoods.org/lessons/Central Asia and Eastern Europe/ SLLPC [accessed 9/1/2013]

Jones, L. and Sidell, M. (eds) (1997) *The Challenge of Promoting Health: Exploration and Action* (London: MacMillan)

Jones, L., Sidell, M. and Douglas, J. (eds) (2002) *The Challenge of Promoting Health: Exploration and Action*. 2nd edn (London: Palgrave Macmillan)

Joubert, N., Taylor, L. and Williams, I. (1996). *Mental Health Promotion: The Time Is Now* (Ottawa: Mental Health Promotion Unit, Health Canada)

Kant, I. (2004) *Kritik av det praktiska förnuftet [Kritik der praktischen Vernunft]* (Stockholm: Thales)

Kashefi, E. and Mort, M. (2004) '"Grounded Citizens" Juries: A Tool for Health Activism?' *Health Expectations*, 7 (4): pp. 290–302

Keleher, H., Mac Dougall, C. and Murphy, B. (2007) *Understanding Health Promotion* (Melbourne: Oxford University Press)

Kelly, J.A. *et al.* (1992) 'Community AIDS/HIV Risk Reduction: The Effects of Endorsements by Popular People in Three Cities', *American Journal of Public Health*, 82 (11): pp. 1483–1489

Kendall, S. (ed) (1998) *Health and Empowerment: Research and Practice* (London: Arnold)

Kieffer, C.H. (1984) 'Citizen Empowerment: A Development Perspective', *Prevention in Human Services*, 3: pp. 9–36

Kohl III, H. and Murray, T. (2012) *Foundations of Physical Activity and Public Health* (Illinois: Human Kinetics)

Kotler, P. (2000) *Marketing Management* (New Jersey: Prentice Hall)

Kroeker, C. (1995) 'Individual, Organizational and Societal Empowerment: A Study of the Processes in a Nicaraguan Agricultural Cooperative', *American Journal of Community Psycology*, 23 (5): pp. 749–764

Kumpfer, K. *et al.* (1993) 'Leadership and Team Effectiveness in Community Coalitions for the Prevention of Alcohol and Other Drug Abuse', *Health Education Research: Theory and Practice,* 8 (3): pp. 359–374

Labonte, R. (1996) Community Development in the Public Health Sector: The Possibilities of an Empowering Relationship between the State and Civil Society', *PhD Thesis* (Toronto: York University)

Labonte, R. (1998) *A Community Development Approach to Health Promotion: A Background Paper on Practice Tensions, Strategic Models and Accountability Requirements for Health Authority Work on the Broad Determinants of Health* (Edinburgh: Health Education Board for Scotland)

Labonte, R. and Laverack, G. (2001a) 'Capacity Building in Health Promotion, Part 1: For Whom? And for What Purpose?' *Critical Public Health,* 11 (2): pp. 111–127

Labonte, R. and Laverack, G. (2001b) 'Capacity Building in Health Promotion, Part 2: Whose Use? And with What Measure? *Critical Public Health,* 11 (2): pp. 129–138

Labonte, R. and Laverack, G. (2008) *Health Promotion in Action: From Local to Global Empowerment* (Basingstoke: Palgrave Macmillan)

Labonte, R. and Robertson, A. (1996) 'Delivering the Goods, Showing our Stuff: The Case for a Constructivist Paradigm for Health Promotion and Research', *Health Education Quarterly,* 23 (4): pp. 431–447

Lalonde, M. (1974) *A New Perspective on the Health of Canadians* (Ottawa: Department of Health and Welfare Canada)

Lancet (2012) 'Patient Empowerment – Who Empowers Whom?' *The Lancet,* 379 (9827): p. 1677

LaVeist, T. (2005) *Minority Populations and Health: An Introduction to Health Disparities in the US* (San Francisco, CA: Jossey-Bass)

Laverack, G. (1999) 'Addressing the Contradiction Between Discourse and Practice in Health Promotion', *Unpublished PhD Thesis* (Melbourne: Deakin University)

Laverack, G. (2001) 'An Identification and Interpretation of the Organizational Aspects of Community Empowerment', *Community Development Journal,* 36 (2): pp. 40–52

Laverack, G. (2004) *Health Promotion Practice: Power and Empowerment* (London: Sage Publications)

Laverack, G. (2005) *Public Health: Power, Empowerment and Professional Practice* (Basingstoke: Palgrave Macmillan)

Laverack, G. (2007) *Health Promotion Practice: Building Empowered Communities* (Maidenhead: Open University Press)

Laverack, G. (2009) *Public Health: Power, Empowerment and Professional Practice,* 2nd edn (Basingstoke: Palgrave Macmillan)

Laverack, G. (2010) 'Editorial. IUHPE', *Global Health Promotion*, 17 (2): pp. 1–2

Laverack, G. (2012) 'Debate: Health Activism', Health Promotion International, 27 (4): pp. 429–434

Laverack, G. (2012a) 'Where Are the Champions of Global Health Promotion? Commentary', *Global Health Promotion*, 19 (2): pp. 63–65

Laverack, G. (2013) *Health Activism: Foundations and Strategies* (London: Sage Publications)

Laverack, G. and Dao, H.D. (2003) 'Transforming Information, Education and Communication in Vietnam', *Health Education*, 103 (6): pp. 363–369

Laverack, G. and Labonte, R. (2000) 'A Planning Framework for the Accommodation of Community Empowerment Goals within Health Promotion Programming', *Health Policy and Planning*, 15 (3): pp. 255–262

Lee, K. (2003) *Globalization and Health: An Introduction* (Basingstoke: Palgrave Macmillan)

Lee, N. and Kotler, P. (2011) *Social Marketing: Influencing Behaviours for Good*. 4th edn (London: Sage Publications)

Lerner, M. (1986) *Surplus Powerlessness* (Oakland: The Institute for Labour and Mental Health)

Levine, B. (2008) *The Art of Lobbying: Building Trust and Selling Policy* (Washington: CQ Press)

Lewis, D. (2003) 'Civil Society. Encyclopedia of Community', *SAGE Publications*, http://www.sage-ereference.com/vi ew/community/n75. xml. [accessed 5/12/2011]

Libby, P. (2011) *The Lobbying Strategy Handbook: 10 Steps to Advancing Any Cause Effectively* (London: Sage Publications)

Lin, N. (2000) 'Inequality in Social Capital', *Contemporary Sociology*, 29: pp. 785–795

Lindquist, E.A. (2001) 'Discerning Policy Influence: Framework for a Strategic Evaluation of IDRC-Supported Research', www.idrc.ca/uploads/user-S/10359907080discerning_policy.pdf [accessed 3/2/2013]

Lindstrom, B. and Eriksson, M. (2005) 'Salutogenesis', *Journal of Epidemiology and Community Health*, 59 (6): pp. 440–442

Lindström, B. and Eriksson, M. (2010) 'The Hitchhiker's Guide to Salutogenesis: Salutogenic Pathways to Health Promotion', *Fokhalsan Health Promotion Research Report 2* (Helsinki: Finland)

Loue, S., Lloyd, L.S. and O'shea, D.J. (2003) *Community Health Advocacy* (New York: Kluwer Academic/Plenum Publishers)

Lund, C. *et al.* (2011) 'Poverty and Mental Disorder: Breaking the Cycle in Low-Income and Middle-Income Countries', *The Lancet*, 378: pp. 1502–1514

Lustig, S. (2012) *Advocacy Strategies for Health and Mental Health Professionals: From Patients to Policies* (New York: Springer Publishing Company)

Mackie, G. (1996) 'Ending Footbinding and Infibulation: A Convention Account', *American Sociological Review*, 61 (6): pp. 999–1017

MacPherson, D.W. and Gushulak, B.D. (2004) 'Global Migration Perspectives: Global Commission on International Migration', (Geneva), Report Number 7. October 2004

McGrath, C. (2007) 'Coalition Building' in G.L. Andersen and K.G. Herr (eds), *Encyclopedia of Activism and Social Justice* (London: Sage Publications)

McGrath, C. (2007a) 'Lobbying' in G.L. Andersen and K.G. Herr (eds), *Encyclopedia of Activism and Social Justice* (London: Sage Publications)

McKinlay, J.B. (1979) 'A Case for Refocusing Upstream: The Political Economy of Illness' in E.G. Jaco (ed), *Patients, Physicians and Illness* (New York: The Free Press)

McLeod, J. and Mcleod, J. (2011) *A Practical Guide for Counsellors and Helping Professionals* (Maidenhead: Open University Press)

McQueen, D. and de Salazar, L. (2011) 'Health Promotion, the Ottawa Charter and "Developing Personal Skills": A Compact History of 25 Years', *Health Promotion International*, 26 (Supplement 2): pp. 194–201

Mad Pride (2013) http://www.madpride.org.uk/. [accessed 31/1/2013]

Maibach, E.W., Rothschild, M.L. and Novelli, W.D. (2002) 'Social Marketing' in K. Glanz, B.K. Rimer and F.M. Lewis (eds), *Health Behavior and Health Education: Theory, Research, and Practice*. 3rd edn (San Franciso, CA: Jossey-Bass), pp. 347–361

Marlatt, G.A. and Witkiewitz, K. (2010) 'Update on Harm-Reduction Policy and Intervention Research', *Annual Review Clinical Psychology*, 6: pp. 591–606

Marlatt, G.A., Larimer, M.E. and Witkiewitz, K. (2011) *Harm Reduction. Pragmatic Strategies for Managing High-Risk Behaviors*. 2nd edn (London: Guildford Press)

Marmot, M., Allen, J. and Goldblatt, P. (2010) 'A Social Movement, Based on Evidence, to Reduce Inequalities in Health', *Social Science and Medicine*, 71: pp. 1254–1258

Marmot, M. and Wilkinson, R.G. (2005) *Social Determinants of Health* (Oxford: Oxford University Press)

Marshall, G. (1998) *A Dictionary of Sociology* (London: Oxford University Press)

Martin, B. (2007) 'Activism, Social and Political' in G.L. Andersen and K.G. Herr (eds), *Encyclopedia of Activism and Social Justice* (London: Sage Publications)

Metoyer, A.B. (2007) 'Natural Childbirth Movement' in G.L. Andersen and K.G. Herr (eds), *Encyclopedia of Activism and Social Justice* (London: Sage Publications)

Micheletti, M. and Stolle, D. (2007) 'Mobilizing Consumers to Take Responsibility for Global Social Justice', *Annals of the American Academy of Political and Social Science*, 611: pp. 157–175

Minkler, M. (1989) 'Health Education, Health Promotion and the Open Society: An Historical Perspective,' *Health Education Quarterly*, 16: pp. 17–30

Monti, P.M. *et al.* (1999) 'Brief Intervention for Harm Reduction and Alcohol Practices in Older Adolescents in a Hospital Emergency Department,' *Journal of Counseling and Clinical Psychology*, 76 (6): pp. 989–994

Morriss, P. (1987) *Power: A Philosophical Analysis* (New York: St. Martin's Press)

Mouy, B. and Barr, A. (2006) 'The Social Determinants of Health: Is There a Role for Health Promotion Foundations?' *Health Promotion Journal of Australia.*, 17 (3): pp. 189–195

Naidoo, J. and Wills, J. (2009) *Foundations for Health Promotion*. 3rd edn (Edinburgh: Bailliere and Tindall)

Nathanson, C. and Hopper, K. (2010) 'The Marmot Review-Social Revolution by Stealth', *Social Science and Medicine*, 71: pp. 1237–1239

The National Institute for Health and Clinical Excellence, http://www.nice.org.uk. [accessed 15/3/2013]

National Iodine Deficiency Disorder Control Program (2000) 'IDD Surveillance in Vietnam the Year 2000' (Ministry of Health. Hanoi. Vietnam)

Navarro, V. (2009) 'What We Mean by Social Determinants of Health'. *Global Health Promotion*, 16 (1): pp. 5–16.

Navarro, V. and Shi, L. (2001) 'The Political Context of Social Inequalities and Health', *Social Science and Medicine*, 52: pp. 481–491

Neilson, S. (2001) 'IDRC-supported Research and its Influence on Public Policy. Knowledge Utilization and Public Policy Processes: A Litera ture Review', IDRC Evaluation Unit, http://idrinfo.idrc.ca/archive/corpdocs/117145/litreview_E.html

Network of Public Health Observatories. (2013) http://www.apho.org.uk/. [accessed 22/1/2013]

Network of Health Promotion Foundations. http://www.who.int/health-promotion/areas/foundations/en/index.html

New South Wales Government (2013) Health, www.health.nsw.gov.au/publichealth/healthpromotion/evidence/. [accessed 21/1/2013]

Nip, J. (2004) 'The Queer Sisters and Its Electronic Bulletin Board: A Study of the Internet for Social Movement Mobilization'. *Information, Communication & Society*, 7: pp. 23–49.

Noar, S.M. and Grant-Harrington, N. (2012) *eHealth Applications: Promising Strategies for Behaviour Change* (New York: Routledge)

Nomura, S. and Ishida, T. (2003) 'Online Communities', [Computerized Tools for Encyclopedia of Community: Sage Publications], http://www.sage-ereference.com/view/community/n362.xml. [accessed 5/12/2011]

Nutbeam, D. (2000) 'Health Literacy as a Public Health Goal: A Challenge for Contemporary Health Education and Communication Strategies into the 21st Century', *Health Promotion International*, 15 (3): pp. 259–267

Nutbeam, D. and Bauman, A (2006) *Evaluation in a Nutshell* (Sydney, Australia: McGraw-Hill Book Company)

Nutbeam, D., Harris, E. and Wise, M. (2010) *Theory in a Nutshell: A Practical Guide to Health Promotion Theories*. 3rd edn (Maidenhead: McGraw-Hill)

Oakes, M. and Kaufman, J. (2006) *Methods in Social Epidemiology* (San Francisco, CA: Jossey Bass)

Ogden, J. (2002) *Health and the Construction of the Individual: A Social Study of Social Science* (London: Routledge)

Osborne, H. (2011) *Health Literacy: A to Z*. 2nd edn (Boston, MA: Jones and Bartlett Learning)

Pakulski, J. (1991) *Social Movements: The Politics of Moral Protest* (Sydney: Longman)

Parker, R. and Sommer, M. (2011) *Handbook in Global Public Health* (Abingdon: Routledge)

Patient Concern (2012) http://www.patientconcern.org.uk/. [accessed 15/1/2012]

Patient UK (2012) www.patient.co.uk. [accessed 21/5/2012]

Patients Association (2011) http://www.patients-association.com. [accessed 15/12/2011]

Patton, M.Q. (1997) 'Toward Distinguishing Empowerment Evaluation and Placing it in a Larger Context', *Evaluation Practice*, 18 (2): pp. 147–163

Peoples Health Movement (2012) www.phmovement.org. [accessed 23/2/2012]

Perez, M. and Luquis, R. (2008) *Cultural Competence in Health Education and Health Promotion* (San Francisco, CA: Jossey-Bass)

Perkins, E., Simnett, I. and Wright, L. (1999) *Evidence Based Health Promotion* (London: Wiley)

Pescosolido, B.A. (1991) 'Illness Careers and Network Ties: A Conceptual Approach of Utilization and Compliance' in G. Albrecht and J. Levy (eds), *Advances in Medical Sociology* (Greenwich, CT: JAI Press), pp. 161–184

Petersen, A.R. (1994) 'Community Development in Health Promotion: Empowerment or Regulation?' *Australian Journal of Public Health*, 18 (2): pp. 213–217

Peterson, C., Maier, S. and Seligman, M. (1995) *Learned Helplessness: A Theory for the Age of Personal Control* (New York: Oxford University Press)

Photo-voice (2013) 'Social Change through Photography', www.photovoice.org. [accessed 5/3/2013]

Pless, B. and Hagel, B. (2005) 'Injury Prevention: A Glossary of Terms', *Journal of Epidemiology and Community Health,* 59 (3): pp. 182–185

Plested, B., Edwards, R. and Jumper-Thurman, P. (2003) *Community Readiness – The Key to Successful Change* (The Tri-ethnic Center for Prevention Research, Sage Hall; Fort Collins, CO: Colorado State University)

Plows, A. (2007) 'Strategies and Tactics in Social Movements' in G.L. Andersen and K.G. Herr (eds), *Encyclopedia of Activism and Social Justice* (London: Sage Publications)

Potvin, L. (2009) 'Yes! More Research is Needed; But Not Just Any Research', *International Journal of Public Health,* 54: pp. 127–128

Public Health Agency of Canada (PHAC) (2013) 'Glossary of Terms', http://www.phac-aspc.gc.ca/php-psp/ccph-cesp/glos-eng.php#h. [accessed 21/1/2013]

Puska, P. *et al.* (eds) (1995) *The North Karelia Project: 20 Year Results and Experiences* (Helsinki: The National Public Health Institute)

Putnam, R.D. (1993) *Making Democracy Work: Civic Traditions in Modern Italy* (Princeton, NJ: Princeton University Press)

Raffle, A.E. and Muir Gray, J.A. (2007) *Screening: Evidence and Practice* (Oxford: Oxford University Press)

Raphael, D. (2000) 'The Question of Evidence in Health Promotion', *Health Promotion International,* 15 (4): pp. 355–367

Rathgeber, E. (2009) 'Research Partnerships in International Health: Capitalizing on Opportunity', Commissioned paper prepared for WHO-TDR meeting on research partnerships, Berlin, Germany

Rebien, C.C. (1996) 'Participatory Evaluation of Development Assistance: Dealing with Power and Facilitative Learning', *Evaluation,* 2 (2): pp. 151–171

renewal.net (2008) 'Resolving Differences-building Communities and Aik Saath: Conflict Resolution Peer Group Facilitators,' Renewal.net case studies, http://www.renewal.net/Documents/RNET/. [accessed 29/4/2008]

Renkert, S. and Nutbeam, D. (2001) 'Opportunities to Improve Maternal Health Literacy through Antenatal Education: An Explanatory Study', *Health Promotion International,* 16 (4): pp. 381–388

Rifkin, S.B. (1990) *Community Participation in Maternal and Child Health/ Family Planning Programmes* (Geneva: World Health Organization)

Rifkin, S.B. and Pridmore, P. (2001) *Partners in Planning: Information, Participation and Empowerment* (London: MacMillan Education)

Ritter, A. and Cameron, J. (2006) 'A Review of the Efficacy and Effectiveness of Harm Reduction Strategies for Alcohol, Tobacco and Illicit Drugs', *Drug Alcohol Rev.*, 25 (6): pp. 611–624

Rissel, C. (1994) 'Empowerment: The Holy Grail of Health Promotion?' *Health Promotion International*, 9 (1): pp. 39–47

Roberts, J.M. (2004) *Alliances, Coalitions and Partnerships: Building Collaborative Organisations* (Gabriola Island, Canada: New Society Publishers)

Robertson, J., Catanzarite, J. and Hong, L. (2010) *Peer Health Education: Concepts and Content* (San Diego, CA: University Readers)

Rohlinger, D.A. and Brown, J. (2009) 'Democracy, Action and the Internet after 9/11', *American Behavioural Scientist*, 53 (1): pp. 133–150

Rootman, I., Goodstadt, M., Hyndman, B., McQueen, D., Potvin, L., Springett, J. and Ziglio, E. (2001) *Evaluation in Health Promotion: Principles and Perspectives*. Series number 92 (Copenhagen: WHO European Office)

Rowitz, L. (2013) *Public Health Leadership*. 3rd edn (Boston, MA: Jones and Bartlett Learning)

Rychetnik, L. and Wise, M. (2004) 'Advocating Evidence-based Health Promotion: Reflections and a Way Forward', *Health Promotion International*, 19 (2): pp. 247–257

Sabo, D. and Gordon, D. (1995) *Men's Health and Illness: Gender, Power and the Body* (London: Sage Publications)

Salmon, P. and Hall, G.M. (2004) 'Patient Empowerment or the Emperor's New Clothes', *Journal of the Royal Society of Medicine*, 97 (2): pp. 53–56

Sargent, C.F. and Brettell, C. (1996) *Gender and Health: An International Perspective* (New Jersey: Prentice Hall)

Schiavo, R. (2007) *Health Communication: From Theory to Practice* (San Francisco, CA: Jossey-Bass)

Scrambler, G. (1987) 'Habermas and the Power of Medical Expertise' in G. Scrambler (ed), *Sociological Theory and Medical Sociology* (New York: Methuen Press)

Scrimgeour, D. (1997) *Community Control of Aboriginal Health Services in the Northern Territory* (Darwin: Menzies School of Health Research)

Scriven, A. and Hodgins, M. (2011) *Health Promotion Settings: Principles and Practice* (London: Sage Publications)

Scott, J. (2001) *Power* (Cambridge, UK: Polity Press)

Seedhouse, D. (1997) *Health Promotion: Philosophy, Prejudice and Practice* (New York/Toronto: Wiley & Sons)

Seidman, S. and Wagner, D.G. (eds) (1992) *Postmodernism and Social Theory: The Debate over General Theory* (Oxford: Blackwell)

Seiter, R.H. and Gass, J.S. (2010) *Persuasion, Social Influence, and Compliance Gaining*. 4th edn (Boston, MA: Allyn & Bacon)

Sharma, M., Atri, A. and Branscum, P. (2011) *Foundations of Mental Health Promotion* (Boston, MA: Jones and Bartlett Learning)

Sharma, M. and Romas, J.A. (2010) *Theoretical Foundations of Health Education and Health Promotion* (Boston, MA: Jones and Bartlett Learning)

Simons-Morton, B., McLeroy, K.C. and Wendel, M.L. (2011) *Behavior Theory in Health Promotion Practice and Research* (New York: Jones and Bartlett Learning)

Simpson, G.E. and Yinger, J.M. (1965) *Racial and Cultural Minorities* (New York: Harper and Row)

Skrentny, J. (2004) *The Minority Rights Revolution* (Boston, MA: Belkap Press of Harvard University Press)

Smith, B., Tang, K.C. and Nutbeam, D. (2006) *Who Health Promotion Glossary: New Terms. Health Promotion International*, 21 (4): pp. 340–345

Smith, J. and Robertson, S. (2008) 'Men's Health Promotion: A New Frontier in Australia and the UK?' *Health Promotion International*, 23 (3): pp. 283–289

Smith, R. (2002) 'The Discomfort of Patient Power', *British Medical Journal*, 324: pp. 497–498

Smithies, J. and Webster, G. (1998) *Community Involvement in Health* (Aldershot, England: Ashgate Publishing)

Staggenborg, S. (2010) *Social Movements* (Oxford: Oxford University Press)

Starhawk, M.S. (1990) *Truth or Dare. Encounters with Power, Authority and Mystery* (New York: HarperCollins)

Stewart, M.A. *et al.* (2003) *Patient Centred Medicine: Transforming the Clinical Method*. 2nd edn (Oxford: Radcliffe Medical Publications)

Sturgeon, S. (2007) 'Promoting Mental Health as an Essential Aspect of Health Promotion', *Health Promotion International*, 21 (Supplement 1): pp. 36–41

Swift, C. and Levin, G. (1987) 'Empowerment: An Emerging Mental Health Technology', *Journal of Primary Prevention*, 8 (1 and 2): pp. 71–94

Swinburn, B., Eggar, G. and Raza, F. (1999) 'Dissecting Obesogenic Environments: The Development and Application of a Framework for Identifying and Prioritizing Environmental Interventions for Obesity', *Preventive Medicine*, 29 (6): pp. 563–570

Syme, L. (1997) 'Individual vs Community Interventions in Public Health Practice: Some Thoughts about a New Approach', *Vichealth Letter*, July, (2): pp. 2–9

Taylor, L., Gowman, N. and Quigley, K. (2003) *Evaluating Health Impact Assessment* (London: Health Development Agency)

Tengland, P. (2007) 'Empowerment: A Goal or a Means for Health Promotion?' *Medicine, Health Care and Philosophy*, 10: pp. 197–207

Thai Health Promotion Foundation. http://en.thaihealth.or.th/

Tilly, C. (2004) *Social Movements, 1768–2004* (Boulder, CO: Paradigm Press)

Tilly, C. and Lesley, J. (2012) *Social Movements, 1768–2012* (Boulder, CO: Paradigm Press)

Tones, K. and Green, J. (2004) *Health Promotion: Planning and Strategies* (London: Sage Publications)

Tones, K. and Tilford, S. (2001) *Health Education: Effectiveness, Efficiency and Equity.* 3rd edn (Cheltenham: Nelson Thornes)

Turner, B.S. and Samson, C. (1995) *Medical Power and Social Knowledge* (London: Sage Publications)

UK Screening Portal (2013) 'UK National Screening Committee'. http://www.screening.nhs.uk/ [accessed 27/2/2013]

UNDP (2002) 'Communication Behaviour Change Tools', *Entertainment-Education,* Vol. 1 (New York: UNDP), pp. 1–6

UNICEF (1999) 'A Manual on Health Promotion. Water, Environment and Sanitation Technical Guidelines', Series 6 (UNICEF: New York)

UNICEF (2001) 'Effective Information, Education and Communication in Vietnam' (UNICEF Hanoi, Vietnam)

UNICEF (2001a) *Beyond Child Labour: Affirming Rights* (New York: UNICEF)

UNICEF (2013) 'Peer Education', http://www.unicef.org/lifeskills/index_12078.html. [accessed 21/1/2013]

Usher, C.L. (1995) 'Improving Evaluability through Self-Evaluation', *Evaluation Practice,* 16 (1): pp. 59–68

Valente, T.W. (2002) *Evaluating Health Promotion Programs* (Oxford: Oxford University Press)

Van Ryn, M. and Heany, C. (1992) 'What's the Use of Theory?' *Health Education Quarterly,* 19 (3): pp. 315–330

Walker, K., MacBride, A. and Vachon, M. (1977) 'Social Support Networks and the Crisis of Bereavement', *Social Science and Medicine,* 11: pp. 35–41

Wallack, L.M. *et al.* (1993) *Media Advocacy and Public Health* (London: Sage Publications)

Wallerstein, N. (1992) 'Powerlessness, Empowerment and Health: Implications for Health Promotion Programs', *American Journal of Health Promotion,* 6 (3): pp. 197–205

Wallerstein, N. and Bernstein, E. (1988) 'Empowerment Education: Freire's Ideas Adapted to Health Education', *Health Education Quarterly,* 15 (4): pp. 379–394

Wang, C. *et al.* (1998) 'Photovoice as a Participatory Health Promotion Strategy', *Health Promotion International,* 13 (1): pp. 75–86

Wasserman, S. and Faust. K.B. (1994) *Social Network Analysis: Methods and Applications* (New York: Cambridge University Press)

Watts, D. (2007) *Pressure Groups* (Edinburgh: Edinburgh University Press)

Weatherburn, D. (2009) 'Dilemmas in Harm Minimization', *Addiction,* 104 (3): pp. 335–339

Weinreich, N. (2010) *Hands-On Social Marketing: A Step by Step Guide to Designing Change for Good.* 2nd edn (London: Sage Publications)

Werner, D. (1988) 'Empowerment and Health', *Contact, Christian Medical Commission,* 102: pp. 1–9

Wasserman, S. and Faust, K.B. (1994) *Social Network Analysis: Methods and Applications* (New York: Cambridge University Press)

White, H.C. (1992) *Identity and Control: A Structured Theory of Social Action* (Princeton, NJ: Princeton University Press)

Wilkinson, R.G. (ed) (2003) *Social Determinants of Health: The Solid Facts.* 2nd edn (Copenhagen, Denmark: WHO Regional Office for Europe)

Woolf, S., Jonas, S. and Kaplan-Liss, E. (2007) *Health Promotion and Disease Prevention in Clinical Practice* (Philadelphia: Lippincott Williams and Wilkins)

World Health Organization (1978) *Alma Ata Declaration* (Geneva: World Health Organization)

World Health Organization (1986) *Ottawa Charter for Health Promotion* (Geneva: World Health Organization)

World Health Organization (1988) *Conference Statement. The Adelaide Recommendations,* www.who.int/hpr

World Health Organization (1991) *Sundsvall Statement on Supportive Environments for Health* (Geneva: World Health Organization)

World Health Organization (EURO) (1991) *Budapest Declaration on Health Promoting Hospitals* (Copenhagen: World Health Organization)

World Health Organization Regional Office for the Western Pacific (1995) *The Yanuca Island Declaration* (Manila: World Health Organization)

World Health Organization (1997) *The Jakarta Declaration on Leading Health Promotion into the 21st Century* (Geneva: World Health Organization)

World Health Organization (1997a) *Promoting Health through Schools: Report of a WHO Expert Committee on Comprehensive School Health Education and Promotion* (Geneva. Technical Report Series No 870)

World Health Organization (1998) *The Health promotion Glossary* (Geneva: World Health Organization)

World Health Organization (2000) *Mexico Global Conference for Health Promotion* (Geneva: World Health Organization)

World Health Organization (2001) *Strengthening Mental Health Promotion.* Fact sheet 220 (Geneva: World Health Organization)

World Health Organization (2002) *The World Health Report 2002 – Reducing Risks, Promoting Healthy Life* (Geneva: World Health Organization)

World Health Organization (2002) *Statement from the 2nd Meeting of the International Network of Health Promoting Foundations.* Bangkok. 4–6 March 2002 (Geneva. World Health Organization)

World Health Organization (2004) *The World Health Report 2003: Shaping the Future* (Geneva: World Health Organization)

World Health Organization (2005) *The Bangkok Charter for Health Promotion in a Globalized World,* 6th Global Conference on Health Promotion (Geneva. World Health Organization)

World Health Organization (2008) *Closing the gap in a generation. Commission on Social determinants of Health. Final Report* (Geneva: World Health Organization), www.who.int/social_determinants. [accessed 6/5/2012]

World Health Organization (2008a) *The World Health Report. Primary Health Care (Now more than ever)* (Geneva: World Health Organization)

World Health Organization (2009) *The Nairobi 7th Global Conference on Health Promotion* (Geneva: World Health Organization)

World Health Organization (2009a) *Milestones in Health Promotion: Statements from Global Conferences* (Geneva: World Health Organization)

World Health Organization (2013) *Chronic Diseases and Health Promotion* (Geneva: WHO), http://www.who.int/chp/en/. [accessed 21/1/2013]

World Health Organization (2013a) *Women's Health* (Geneva: World Health Organization), http://www.who.int/topics/womens_health/en/. [accessed 21/1/2013]

Wright, E.R. (1997) 'The Impact of Organizational Factors on Mental Health Professionals' Involvement with Families', *Psychiatric Services,* 48: pp. 921–927

Wright, J. (2001) 'Assessing Health Needs' in D. Pencheon, J.A. Muir Gray, C. Guest and D. Melzer (eds), *Oxford Handbook of Public Health Practice* (Oxford: Oxford University Press), pp. 38–47

Wright, K., Sparks, L. and O'Hair, D. (2012) *Health Communication in the 21st Century.* 2nd edn (London: Wiley Blackwell)

Wrong, D.H. (1988) *Power: Its Forms, Bases and Uses* (Chicago, IL: The University of Chicago Press)

Yeatman, A. (1998) *Activism and the Policy Process* (Sydney: Allen & Unwin)

Young, L. and Everitt, J. (2004) *Advocacy Groups* (Vancouver, BC: University of British Columbia Press)

Zakus, J.D.L. and Lysack, C.L. (1998) 'Revisiting Community Participation', *Health Policy and Planning,* 13 (1): pp. 1–12

Zajda, J., Majhanovich, S. and Rust, V. (2006) *Education and Social Justice* (London: Springer)

index

Note: Main entries are in bold and numbers in bold refer to quick access for a definition.